ETHICAL DILEMMAS & NURSING PRACTICE

Fifth Edition

ETHICAL DILEMMAS & NURSING PRACTICE

Anne J. Davis RN, PhD, DSc (hon), FAAN

Professor Emerita
School of Nursing
University of California, San Francisco
Nagano College of Nursing
Komagane, Nagano, Japan

Marsha D. Fowler, PhD, MDiv, MS, RN, FAAN

Professor of Ethics and Spirituality
Azusa Pacific University
Azusa, California

Mila Ann Aroskar, EdD, DSc (hon)

Faculty Associate Emerita
Center for Bioethics
University of Minnesota
Minneapolis, Minnesota

Pearson

Boston Columbus Indianapolis New York San Francisco Upper Saddle River
Amsterdam Cape Town Dubai London Madrid Milan Munich Paris Montreal Toronto
Delhi Mexico City Sao Paulo Sydney Hong Kong Seoul Singapore Taipei Tokyo

Publisher: Julie Alexander
Assistant to Publisher: Regina Bruno
Editor-in-Chief: Maura Connor
Assistant to Editor-in-Chief: Marion Gottlieb
Executive Editor: Pamela Fuller
Editorial Assistant: Lisa Pierce
Director of Marketing: Karen Allman
Senior Marketing Manager: Francisco
  Del Castillo
Marketing Specialist: Michael Sirinides

Marketing Assistant: Crystal Gonzalez
Art Director: Jayne Conte
Cover Designer: Margaret Kenselaar
Media Director: Allyson Graesser
Lead Media Project Manager: Rachel Collett
Production Manager: Fran Russello
Full-Service Project Management: Sadagoban
  Balaji/Integra Software Services, Pvt. Ltd
Printer/Binder: King Printing Co., Inc.
Text Font: 10/12, Garamond

Credits and acknowledgments for materials borrowed from other sources and reproduced, with permission, in this textbook appear on appropriate page within text.

Library of Congress Cataloging-in-Publication Data

Davis, Anne J.,
  Ethical dilemmas & nursing practice/Anne J. Davis, Marsha D. Fowler,
Mila Ann Aroskar.—5th ed.
     p.; cm.
  Rev. ed. of: Ethical dilemmas and nursing practice/Anne J. Davis . . . et al.]. 4th ed. c1997.
  Includes bibliographical references and index.
  ISBN-13: 978-0-13-092973-0 (alk. paper)
  ISBN-10: 0-13-092973-5 (alk. paper)
  1. Nursing ethics.   I. Fowler, Marsha Diane Mary   II. Aroskar, Mila A.   III. Ethical dilemmas
and nursing practice.   IV. Title.   V. Title: Ethical dilemmas and nursing practice.
[DNLM: 1. Ethics, Nursing. WY 85 D261ed 2010]
RT85.D33 2010
174.2—dc22

                                                                            2009018775

  6 7 8 9 10   V0CR   15 14 13 12

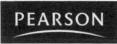

Prentice Hall
is an imprint of

www.pearsonhighered.com

ISBN 10:   0-13-092973-5
ISBN 13: 978-0-13-092973-0

REVIEWERS

DeAnn L. Ambroson, PhD, RN, LMSW, COI
Professor
Allen College

Glenda Avery, PhD, APRN-BC
Associate Professor
School of Nursing, Troy University

Sarah J. Breier, PhD, RN
Associate Director/Assistant Professor
Sinclair School of Nursing, University of Missouri, Columbia

Diane C. Bridge, BSN, MSN
Assistant Professor of Nursing
Liberty University

Gail E. Bromley, PhD, RN
Associate Dean
College of Nursing, Kent State University

Sheila Cannon, PhD, APRN, BC
Assistant Professor of Nursing
University of Massachusetts, Boston

Peggy N. Flannigan, PhD, RN
Associate Professor
Bradley University

Joan Garity, EdD, RN
Associate Professor
College of Nursing and Health Sciences, University of Massachusetts, Boston

Karen Kovach, BSN, RN
PhD Candidate/Teaching Assistant
School of Nursing, University of Pittsburgh

Jeanne M Maiden, RN, CNS, PhD
Associate Professor
Point Loma Nazarene University

Carol A. Mannahan, EdD, RN, CNAA-BC
Executive Director, Leadership Development
College of Nursing, University of Oklahoma

Diana M. L. Newman, EdD, RN
Professor
School of Nursing, Massachusetts College of Pharmacy and Health Sciences

Polly Royal, RN, DNP
Clinical Assistant Professor
Purdue University

Angela Stone Schmidt, MNSc, RNP, RN
Assistant Professor of Nursing
College of Nursing and Health Professions, Arkansas State University

Erin C. Soucy, MSN, BSN, RN
Interim Director of the Division of Nursing
University of Maine at Fort Kent

Mary S. Tilbury, EdD, RN, NEA-BC
Specialty Coordinator, Leadership and Management
College of Health Sciences, Walden University

Kristi A. Wilkerson, RN, MSN
Nursing Faculty
Southeastern Community College

PREFACE

Marsha Fowler, who contributed to earlier editions, joins me in updating this fifth edition. Mila Aroskar, the earlier coauthor, prepared the chapter on policy, an increasingly important topic in ethics. We all are pleased that readers have found this book helpful since the first edition in 1978. These 30 years have witnessed both change and continuity in the ethical issues facing nurses. This edition reflects nursing's values and ethics in those two contexts. Some chapters have been combined, while others remain the same but updated. A new chapter focuses on selected major trends that present special ethical dilemmas for now and in the future. While the major ethical theoretical frame here is principle-based ethics because it remains the prevailing language used in health science ethical discourse, especially by institutional clinical committees and institutional review boards that review research proposals, alternative approaches are also included. We hope that nurses who read this book will gain more understanding of this ethical approach, including its assumptions, values, concepts, and language, so that they can participate knowledgably in ethical dialogue. We think that nursing input is of vital importance in the deliberation of ethical problems.

We are grateful to many beyond those we can name here. There were many who reviewed this work in manuscript form and we thank them for their thoughtful critique and suggestions. The three authors of this volume share in common having been named Kennedy Fellows in Bioethics in the 1970s. We again thank the Kennedy Foundation for the unparalleled opportunity that the Fellowship afforded us. We also want to most sincerely thank all the people who made this edition possible.

Anne J. Davis,
PhD, DSc (hon), MS, RN, FAAN

Marsha D. Fowler,
PhD, MDiv, MS, RN, FAAN

Mila Ann Aroskar,
EdD, DSc (hon)

CONTENTS

INTRODUCTION TO THE BOOK

This book focuses on nursing ethics and bioethics, both of which are applied subjects. That is, their knowledge base is drawn from several sources outside nursing. The bases used in this book are largely drawn from Western moral philosophy, which has a long history beginning with the Greek philosophers who gave us basic ideas about democracy, the good life, and how we should live with others. American society has also drawn upon various religious traditions for ideas about a just society, what is good, and how we are to respond to the needs of "our neighbor." The combination of these philosophical, religious, and socio-cultural influences has shaped our values, which we often take for granted, sometimes without realizing that our world view is rooted in and informed by these sources. We learn these values about living in the world at home, in school, and from other social institutions. And we learn most of them when we are young, although life experiences can lead people to shift and change in their value structure and moral perspectives. In addition, the legal system in English-speaking countries has also been greatly influenced by these same sources. Legally what constitutes a crime and how the legal system treats people are determined by these ideas that have developed over many centuries. Notions of rights and obligations, harm and good, stem from all these sources: philosophy, religion, the law.

The values in a society can evolve over time when people become more enlightened. For example, not long ago people in Africa were uprooted from their homes and brought to the United States as valued property to be bought and sold. A bloody Civil War in our great-grandmother's lifetime was fought to eliminate slavery. Later, the Civil Rights Movement changed voting rights for this same group. Though racial prejudice is still with us, the world view of many people in the United States has changed, especially since the 1950s. Such changes help us live up to our stated ideals and values. Other examples include the increasing awareness of ageism and sexism in the late 20th century.

Nurses have also witnessed change over recent years with regard to the rights and responsibilities of patients and the limits of medical control in decision making. Some basic values and definitions of rights changed and not too long ago either. This book is about how to use the knowledge sources mentioned above to understand some of these changes and how to think about ethically problematic situations using these ideas. There is nothing more practical than a concept because it allows us to see, understand, and articulate.

This book was written for undergraduate and graduate students, as well as for practicing nurses, most of whom have not had much background in the knowledge base for nursing ethics and bioethics. Since this book is limited to the application of this knowledge, it cannot include detailed discussions about these knowledge sources.

Also while we have mentioned that this book uses essentially Western knowledge bases, it is important to realize that not all people are Western in their values and world view. Their taken-for-granted world may differ significantly from that of a Western-based perspective.

There are other rich world views along with that of the dominant culture. Cross-cultural ethics is a large and important topic mostly beyond the limits of this book. However, to aid you in further exploration of a variety of topics, we have provided a list of readings that can help you to develop a deeper knowledge base beyond what any single book can provide.

CHAPTER 1

Introduction to Ethics and Ethical Dilemmas

DEFINITIONS AND SOURCES OF KNOWLEDGE

Traditionally, philosophy as a body of knowledge has asked and attempted to answer, in a formal and disciplined manner, the great questions of life that any of us might raise with ourselves in our more reflective moments. The branch of philosophy called *ethics*, also referred to as *moral philosophy*, helps us to examine and understand the moral life. It deals with important questions of human conduct that have great relevance to us as individuals and as health professionals. Ethics, as a body of knowledge, has evolved in the Western philosophical tradition since the Golden Age of Greece and deals with the concept of morality and with moral problems and judgments.

The word *ethics*, derived from the Greek term *ethos*, originally meant customs, habitual usages, conduct, and character, and the word *moral*, derived from the Latin *mores*, means customs or habit. Today, in the widest sense, these two words refer to conduct, character, and motives involved in moral acts and include the notion of approval or disapproval of a given conduct, character, or motive that we describe by such words as *good, desirable, right*, and *worthy*, or conversely by such words as *bad, undesirable, wrong, evil*, and *unworthy*. The words *ethical* and *moral* will be used interchangeably in this book.

Often, when we speak of the ethics or morals of an individual or group, we refer to a set of rules or body of principles. Each society, religion, and professional group has its principles or standards of conduct, and as persons concerned with being reasonable in our conduct, we rely on these standards for guidance.

Morality has been defined as a *social* enterprise and not just an invention or discovery by individuals for their own guidance. This social nature of morality is not limited to its being a system governing the relations of one person to others or one's code of action with respect to others. Obviously, morality is social in this sense, but also, as importantly, morality is social in its origins, sanctions, and functions, since we are born into a society that has developed and continues to maintain mores, laws, and ethical codes. As a societal system of regulations, morality shares some similarities with

1

both the law and social convention or etiquette. Convention, as we usually define it, has to do with considerations of taste, appearance, and convenience, and does not deal with matters of crucial social importance. Convention and morality share similarities in that neither is created nor changed by a deliberate judicial, legislative, or executive act. Verbal and nonverbal signs of approval or disapproval, praise or blame, become social sanctions in these instances. In its focus on crucial matters of social importance, such as individual and group rights and obligations, morality shares similarities with the law.

WAYS OF THINKING ABOUT ETHICS

There are several ways to think about ethics, which include normative ethics, practical ethics, and descriptive ethics.

Normative ethics gives us norms we can use to guide our behavior and it can also help us evaluate behavior. For example, nursing's code of ethics states the ethical norms that nurses should use to guide their professional behavior. They can also evaluate their nursing actions and that of others from an ethical perspective using this code.

Practical ethics is the use of ethical theory and analysis to examine moral problems. For example, Nurse A knows that the patient was told, but does not understand his diagnosis and prognoses so she views this as an ethical dilemma involving the principles of respect for autonomy and do no harm.

Descriptive ethics describes people's actual moral beliefs and actions. For example, what, if anything, should Nurse A do about this ethical problem?

The first two of these ways of thinking about ethics are the "oughts" of ethics, while descriptive ethics is what a person may actually do or the "is" of behavior that may or may not be ethical.

ETHICAL THEORIES

In addition to these ways of thinking about ethics, nurses use specific ethical theories although they may not think of their reasoning and actions in this way. Ethical theories, bodies of knowledge that have developed over time, establish our focus of concern, our language of dialogue, and the outcomes of our discourse. These theories can provide a reasoned response to practical questions about how to live, what we should do when facing a dilemma, and how to be a morally good person. Davis, Tschudin, and deRaeve (2006) detail these theories, focusing on what they mean, their limitations, and how they can be used in nursing.

Virtue ethics or character ethics places emphasis on the individual who makes choices and takes actions. A virtue is a moral trait that is praise-worthy, such as compassion, kindness, and so on. Nursing's long interest in and concern about ethics has until recently been with regard to an ethics of virtue. Describing someone as a good nurse, for example, used virtue ethics.

Principle-based ethics asks, what should I do to be ethical in a given situation? In this case, a person would use ethical principles to think through the dilemma. Do no harm, respect for individual autonomy, and do good are among the principles that this theory uses (Beauchamp & Childress, 2001; Davis et al., 2006).

An *Ethics of care* focuses on those traits valued in intimate personal relationships and would include such attributes as compassion, love, sympathy, and trust among others. Since the early 1980s, the ethics of care has been written about predominantly in feminist and nursing sources.

Feminist ethics takes into account the social and cultural structures of politics and power arrangements in everyday moral life. It critiques these same social and cultural structures in relation to even the ethical theory usually used in health care ethics today as well as in the inequalities manifest in professional and personal life.

While at times these ethical theories have been presented as mutually exclusive, in reality we can use a combination of them that helps us explore and reason through different aspects of ethical dilemmas.

In a somewhat simplistic way, we can say that:

- Virtue ethics asks, "What sort of person ought I *be*?"
- Ethical principles (obligation ethics) help us answer the question, "What I ought to *do* when confronted with an ethical problem or dilemma?"
- Ethics of care helps us determine what the nature of a given relationship ought to be.
- Feminist ethics asks about the political and power arrangements and who is advantaged or disadvantaged by them.

In nursing and in life, we need all of these ways to conceptually frame ethical dilemmas. While all of these theoretical approaches to ethics are important and useful, this book in general discusses principle-based ethics more than the other approaches. Principle-based ethics is not without limitations; however, it is this ethics that is predominantly used in clinical situations, clinical ethics committees, research ethics committees, and policy development. Further reading can enhance one's understanding of virtue, feminist, and care ethics (Bayles & Bayles, 1990; Beauchamp & Childress, 2001; Benner, 1994; Davis et al., 2006; Du Bose, Hamel, & O'Connell, 1994; Gilligan, 1993; McIntyre, 1984; Sherman, 1991; Sherwin, 1993; Thomson, 1990). Also see Suggested Additional Readings in Appendix A.

ETHICAL DILEMMAS

Nurses confront many ethical dilemmas in their practice. Such dilemmas include but are not limited to the following: (a) whether and in what way to care for a so-called noncompliant patient, (b) nursing care of a dying patient receiving intensive therapy, (c) the patient asks you to keep in confidence something that is important to share with other health professionals, (d) patient advocacy when the patient and his/her family disagree, (e) not wanting or willing to care for a patient with a highly contagious disease about which little is known, (f) a woman who has had an abortion, and so on. Is there a duty for you to give care to and to care about these patients? What professional values and ethical principles would you use to deal with these clinical situations and potential ethical problems? In any of these situations, do your personal values conflict with your professional obligations? If so, how do you decide what to do ethically? Can you give good nursing care when you have a negative reaction to a patient or when you think that patient has done something morally wrong? What ethical actions might be needed on your part? These are difficult questions best thought about before you face them.

We may be ethical to the extent that our behavior elicits approval and respect from others; however, we still confront moral perplexity and moral doubt. For example, in a situation in which our ethical code guides us to tell the truth, we decide to withhold truthful information because we believe such knowledge will cause psychological harm to the individual hearing it. Such a situation usually confronts health professionals, particularly in caring for terminally ill patients. This example shows that in honoring one moral principle, we can violate another: If we tell the truth, we may risk doing harm to the listener. On the other hand, if we do not tell the truth, we violate the individual's right to information, which affects his or her self-determination. The degree of confidence a community can have in its health professionals remains one critical consideration in the issue of truth telling, the principle of veracity. Although a set of principles and rules is vital to human conduct, it cannot be wholly depended upon for guidance, since it can never be complete enough to anticipate all possible occasions involving moral decisions.

ETHICAL REASONING USING ETHICAL THEORIES

Socrates, the patron saint of Western moral philosophy, in the Crito dialogue argued that we must let reason determine our ethical decisions rather than emotion. To accomplish this, we must have factual information about the situation and keep our minds clear as we deliberate the issue. We need to be aware of our own values and how they influence our definition of and solution to an ethical situation. In addition, values held in common by all nurses must be taken into account. It is not enough to appeal to what people generally think, since they may be wrong, but we must, by informed reasoning, find an answer that we regard as ethically correct. And importantly, according to Socrates, we ought never to do what is morally wrong. The proposal of what we should do in a situation must be viewed according to its right-ness or wrongness as concluded after informed reasoning and not as to what will happen to us as a consequence, or what others will think of us, or how we feel about the situation. In his arguments, Socrates appealed to a general moral rule or principle that, after reflection, he accepted as valid and applicable to particular situations. But in addition, Socrates, aware of the fact that sometimes two or more moral rules apply to the same case but do not lead to the same conclusion, resolved this conflict by determining which rules take precedence over others. Here he went beyond just appealing to rules, since they conflicted with one another, and established what he called basic rules and derivative rules, which rest on the more basic ones. A reason-ing process that establishes basic ethical rules leads to the inevitable question of how ethical principles and judgments are to be justified. A full-fledged discussion develops in moral philosophy when we pass beyond the stage in which we are directed only by traditional rules of conduct, which have limited application to complex ethical situations, and move to a stage where we think critically about an ethical dilemma in ways that allow us to use traditional rules as general principles coupled with ethical reasoning going beyond these traditional rules.

As has been indicated, not all ethical dilemmas can be resolved by an appeal to our common moral rules and principles, and this fact lies at the center of moral philosophy as a field of inquiry. Let it be emphasized, however, that the traditional interest in ethics as a subject matter must not be confused with the practical interest of moral beings. To avoid the mistake of assuming that a knowledge of moral theory is sufficient for the improvement of our moral practice, we must realize that the theoretical interest is concerned with knowing and the practical interest with doing. A moralist engages in reflection and discussion about what is morally right or wrong, good or evil. A moral philosopher thinks and writes about the ways in which moral terms like *right* or *good* are used by moralists when they deliver their moral judgments. If our object is to discover unambiguous answers to ethical dilemmas quickly and effortlessly, most likely we will be bewildered by the complexity of these dilemmas. Furthermore, we will most surely experience disappointment if we expect instant truth, for one does not mine ethical dilemmas as easily as one mines precious metals, but a concern for ethical principles may prove to be the more valuable of the two endeavors.

HEALTH CARE ETHICS

Building on accumulated knowledge, especially from the 17th through the 19th centuries, medical science and technology have progressed triumphantly during recent centuries. In the wake of this progress, two sets of major problems related to optimal health care have arisen: (a) the inadequate distribution and availability, and excessive cost of health care and (b) the danger of becoming so infatuated with the technological dimensions of health care that we cease to question their limitations. Specifically, we can unintentionally lose sight of the axiomatic foundation of health care, which is that human beings cannot be understood in mechanistic terms only. To lose sight of this foundation shows a limited view that could violate that very reason of health care, thereby creating ethical dilemmas.

The health sciences make many demands upon the abilities, special training, and character of their practitioners. One of the most basic of these demands requires that we be guided by moral considerations. Health care ethics, historically also called medical ethics, nursing ethics, biomedical ethics, and more recently, bioethics are normative, practical ethics specific to the health sciences. It raises the question of what is right or what ethically ought to be done in a health care situation when a moral decision is called for. Such situations range from moral decisions in the clinical setting focused on one patient and his or her family to policy decisions such as distribution of resources. Specifically, health care ethics addresses four interrelated areas: (a) clinical practice, (b) allocation of scarce resources, (c) human experimentation, and (d) health policy.

It has been argued that moral considerations in the health sciences do not differ from normal, everyday moral considerations since both use the same virtues and values and moral principles or rules and engage in ethical reasoning. In health care ethics, the difference occurs only in the special situations and issues confronting practitioners. The basic task of health care ethics therefore is not necessarily to discover some new moral principles on which to build a theoretical ethical system or to evolve new approaches to ethical reasoning, but to apply the established virtues and general moral principles or rules. In short, health care ethics is practical, applied ethics. As with general ethics in daily life, we cannot utilize an automatic deductive procedure in health care ethics to arrive at "the" ethical answer, nor can we legitimately expect ethics as a discipline to motivate those of us in the health sciences to be moral or to reprimand us when we are not. Health care ethics does not promote a particular moral life style nor does it campaign for particular life values. Its role has been defined as functioning (a) to sensitize or raise the consciousness of health professionals (and the lay public) concerning ethical issues found in health care settings and policies and (b) to structure the issues so that ethically relevant threads of complex situations can be drawn out and discussed. Health care ethics can illuminate the variety of conflicting ethical principles involved in a particular situation and can isolate pivotal concepts needing definition, clarification, or defense. Principles and theories taken from ethics and applied in the health care arena give us ways to systematically reason through an ethical dilemma. And again, we remind the reader to use Appendix A to gain an in-depth understanding of general ethics and nursing ethics.

HEALTH CARE ETHICS AND THE LAW

Law and ethics in a given society are similar in that they have developed in the same historical, social, cultural, and philosophical soil, but they also differ in some important ways. The relationship between ethics and law is as follows. Actions can be (a) ethical and legal, such as informed consent; (b) unethical and illegal, such as killing; (c) ethical and illegal; and (d) unethical and legal. The latter two possibilities confront health professionals and present the most difficult situations to reason through to a satisfactory solution as they depend on your moral position on certain issues such as physician-assisted suicide and abortion. People would agree on the first two actions in most cases; however, the other two are not always agreed on and often become political in nature.

Because we tend to use the term *right* in a very broad and indiscriminate way, the law can help to limit this term to a workable definition and to a more appropriate meaning. Legal rights are based in the law, whereas ethical rights are based in moral philosophy such as ethical principles and rules. Positive rights mean that one has a *right to* something, and negative rights mean that one has a right to be left alone. Free speech is a positive right, whereas refusing an injection is a negative right, the right to be *left alone*. People have the right to speak and also the right to refuse the injection.

VALUES AND MORAL DEVELOPMENT

Few things in life are value-free. Values are basic to a given way of life and serve to give direction to life. Our values are often similar to our breathing because we take them for granted and are not always aware of them. We do not always examine them but simply accept and act on these values unless we experience difficulty. Much of what goes into our ethical thinking is unarticulated, unspoken values. Most people take moral values and judgments seriously in all aspects of their lives. Furthermore, one's moral convictions are not diminished by the recognition that others have different moral convictions that are taken equally seriously. This reflects the complexities of our multicultural societies and world (Davis et al., 2006).

Intrinsic values or *goods* are those things that are valuable in themselves, such as friendship, while extrinsic values are means to the attainment of other goods such as going to the dentist to have healthy teeth, which is an intrinsic good. These categories are not always mutually exclusive. Education is a good example because it is valuable in itself and it also helps in obtaining employment.

MORAL DEVELOPMENT AND WORLD VIEW

Moral development refers to how and why humans become moral. Several classic studies in psychology conducted by Kohlberg, Milgram, and others have attempted to answer these questions (Kohlberg, 1981; Milgram, 1963).

Later researchers such as Gilligan, Nodding, and others have raised questions about whether there are morally relevant factors in ethics and therefore in health care ethics that need to be taken into account, such as gender, ethnicity, and culture (Gilligan, 1982; Noddings, 1984). Out of these more recent questions, feminist ethics developed to address gender factors and the socio-political context in ethics.

People from different cultures have different views of the world and different values. This fact has led to many questions about how to deal with this reality, especially in our globalized world, that impacts nursing and nurses. How can we reconcile in a nonethnocentric fashion the enforcement of international cross-cultural universal ethics and human rights standards with the protection of cultural diversity? This leads to the larger questions as to whether we have universal values and ethics or whether values and ethics are always embedded in a specific culture. This problem is referred to as the possible conflict between Universal Ethics and Ethical Relativism and both have limitations as ways of thinking about ethics, health care ethics, and nursing ethics. People whose values differ from the dominant cultural values can be perceived as less morally developed because they are judged by a standard that is not their own. This applies not solely to ethnic and racial minorities: women have also been judged as less well developed morally. In a pluralistic society, such as the United States, this is a topic that must be discussed and understood (Davis et al., 2006). See Appendix A for reading on this important and complex topic.

EXAMPLES OF ETHICAL DILEMMAS

As indicated earlier, one of the major difficulties in ethical discourses is that no definite, clear-cut answer exists for all ethical dilemmas. For that reason, critical reflection becomes necessary in any attempt to deal with an ethical dilemma. A dilemma can be defined as (a) a difficult problem seemingly incapable of a satisfactory solution or (b) a situation involving choice between equally unsatisfactory alternatives. Not all dilemmas in life are ethical in nature, but an ethical dilemma does arise when values and moral positions or claims conflict with one another. For example, health professionals ethically ought to prolong life and relieve suffering. But to relieve suffering by medications may shorten the life of a terminally ill patient. Not to give the medicine means that the patient suffers. What should the nurse do to act ethically in this dilemma?

Ethical dilemmas are situations involving conflicting moral positions or claims and give rise to such questions as: What morally should I do? What harm and benefit result from this decision or action? For example, in a situation where moral claims conflict, what one considers good may not necessarily be right. Physician-assisted suicide may be considered a morally good action by some people in a particular situation such as a terminally ill patient with intractable pain, but it may not be considered a positive right for patients and therefore a health professional does not have the duty to perform this action. In a few places, physician-assisted suicide is now legal, but some physicians regard this as unethical and so they say they do not have an ethical duty to engage in this practice.

A less dramatic example but one that may occur more often concerns the conflict between the patient's right to make decisions about his or her medical care, the principle of respect for autonomy, and the health professional's interference with and limitation of that right in the name of health. For example, the violation of patient autonomy by a decision to withhold information about diagnosis and prognoses is justified because disclosing the information might harm the patient and so withholding it is seen to be in the best interests of the patient. What is important to note here is that another person determines the best interest of the patient rather than the patient himself or herself deciding after discussions with appropriate others. This behavior on the part of health professionals has been referred to by some as paternalism, where the health professional's behavior reduces the competent adult patient or the parents of a young patient to something less than decision-making, autonomous individuals.

Another example of conflicting moral claims and the law arises when a hospital applies to the court for an order authorizing the administration of a blood transfusion to a patient who is a Jehovah's Witness. The court usually says in these cases that a competent adult patient has a right, on religious grounds, to refuse a blood transfusion, even if medical opinion is that the patient's decision not to accept blood amounts to the patient's taking his or her own life. If the court determines that the patient was mentally competent when told the necessary information about the blood transfusion and was also competent when he or she made the decision, the court then concludes that this patient must have the final say and that this must necessarily be so in a system of government that gives the greatest possible protection to the individual in the furtherance of his or her own desire. This is a conflict between the patient's religious right to refuse treatment and the doctor's duty to give treatment based on medical judgment.

Because of these and other such dilemmas, a typical patient bill of rights usually contains one section, "Your Right to Decline Treatment." It says that patients do have the right to decline treatment, but it also usually says that if the hospital staff believes that a patient's decision to decline treatment is seriously inconsistent with their ability to provide the patient with adequate care, the patient may be requested to make arrangements elsewhere for health care. This statement clearly draws the ethical dilemma as a conflict between the patient's right to refuse treatment and the hospital staff's duty to provide treatment.

Yet another example of an ethical dilemma is in the clinical research situation. For the purpose of discussion, let us say that a clinical researcher has developed what appears to be an effective therapeutic technique and wishes to test its efficacy on hospital patients who have the disease this technique is designed to cure. For comparative purposes, the patients are divided into two groups by random assignment so that the experimental group will receive the new technique and the control group will receive the currently accepted therapy. After a period of time elapses, the researcher discovers that one group seems to be improving much more rapidly than the other. Regardless of which group improves, we have an ethical dilemma with a conflict between the obligation of the scientist to complete the experiment in order to add to knowledge that can help future patients and the obligation of the clinician to provide present patients with the most effective treatment available. Other research situations call attention to different ethical dilemmas. Research involving children or frail elderly patients, or research with a control group in which the patient is given a placebo are only three examples of such situations.

The preamble to the Constitution of the World Health Organization (WHO) says that the enjoyment of the highest attainable standard of health is one of the fundamental rights of every human being, without distinction on the basis of race, religion, political belief, or economic or social conditions. In the United States, fundamental changes have taken place in the delivery of health care. Managed care and health maintenance organizations (HMOs) are the most recent arrangements, with an emphasis on short hospital stays, outpatient services, and home or community care. It is still the case that many people in the United States do not have health insurance. Indeed, the United States is the only industrialized country that has not defined health care as a right for everyone but rather continues to think of it as a commodity and business. This is a major ethical, political, economic, and social issue under much discussion.

With present economic problems and policies, health and social programs are in danger of being cut or eliminated. The broader ethical question here is, How does one account for societal callousness and indifference when they appear to coexist with a deep and abiding societal concern for others? Perhaps, this conflict arises because in our world view, we see society as operating in a consistent, just manner, so that the bad are punished and the good are rewarded. But is the world really this simple? Or, perhaps the conflict can be explained by the observation that those who are doing well blame the victims, since to do so may relieve them of any felt obligation.

Discussion of numerous ethical dilemmas occurs not only during the development of public policy but continues even after policy becomes enacted into law. The possibility of legislating ethical dilemmas out of the health care scene seems extremely remote. Regardless of the type of health care system, ethical dilemmas will continue to confront health care providers. A recent topic that has received much attention is rationing scarce medical resources. Numerous ethical questions arise, such as, Who should get what when not everyone can get what he or she needs to live? If medical resources are rationed, what criteria should be used to determine their allocation? Would such criteria as age, benefit to patient, contribution to society, and so forth be ethical? Does the present lack of access to health care constitute rationing?

Some people do not like the word "dilemma" and prefer to use such words as "ethical problem or issue." Whatever the words used, they all tell us that we face a situation that requires value clarification, reflection on these values, and possibly actions of an ethical nature.

PROFESSIONAL CODES OF ETHICS IN THE HEALTH SCIENCES

Health care ethics, concerned with rights, duties, and obligations, calls for an interdisciplinary quest for an understanding of professional responsibility. To understand the present situation, an examination of professional codes of ethics should prove fruitful. Although all health professional groups have codes, this discussion focuses mostly on those in nursing. Chapter 3 details the American Nurses Association (ANA) *Code of Ethics*. In addition to the code, ANA has also developed position papers on various important issues. For example, Nursing's *Social Policy Statement*, which defines many aspects of nursing practice, is a classic and should be read by all nurses (ANA, 2004).

In addition, state nurses' associations and specialty groups in nursing have developed standards of practice and position papers on various issues such as patient safety, improving pain management, and nursing education, to mention only a few.

Medical codes of ethics are available online or in medical ethics books and are worthy of our attention but are beyond the scope of this book. Other health-related groups such as the American Public Health Association also have documents that are ethical in nature.

The International Council of Nurses in Geneva updated its *Code of Ethics* in 2005. This document addresses nurses' duties, obligations, and rights. According to this code, nurses have four fundamental responsibilities: to promote health, to prevent illness, to restore health, and to alleviate suffering. It says that inherent in nursing is respect for human rights, including cultural rights, the right to life, choice, and dignity, and the right to be treated with respect. Nursing care is respectful of and unrestricted by considerations of age, color, creed, culture, disability or illness, gender, sexual orientation, nationality, race, or social status. Nurses render health services to the individual, the family, and the community and coordinate their services with those in related groups. The *Code* emphasizes that the nurse's primary professional responsibility is to the people requiring nursing care. To meet this primary ethical obligation, nurses should respect the beliefs, values, and customs of the individual and hold in confidence personal information and use judgment in sharing this.

Each nurse carries personal responsibility for nursing practice and for maintaining competence by continual learning and maintains the highest standards of nursing care possible within the reality of a specific situation. It is necessary for the nurse to use judgment in relation to individual competence when accepting or delegating tasks. The standards of personal conduct that reflect credit upon the profession are essential for the nursing role.

Nurses often through their organizations assume responsibility for initiating and supporting action to meet the health and social needs of the public. They also sustain a cooperative relationship with co-workers in nursing and other specialties and take appropriate action to safeguard the individual when clinical care is endangered by a coworker or any other person.

Nurses play the major role in determining and implementing desirable standards of nursing practice and nursing education and in developing a core of professional knowledge. Through professional organizations, nurses participate in establishing and maintaining equitable social and economic working conditions in nursing.

In order to provide an up-to-date means of professional self-regulation, the ANA periodically revises its code of ethics, originally adopted in 1950 (ANA, 1995). This *Code for Nurses* indicates the nursing profession's acceptance of the responsibility and trust with which it has been invested by society. The requirements of the *Code* may often exceed, but are not less than, those of the law. While violation of the law subjects the nurse to criminal or civil liability, the Association may reprimand, censure, suspend, or expel members from the Association for violation of the *Code*.

Historical Events and Code Development

One tradition that evolved from historical events in the 20th century and led to the development of codes of ethics must be included in any discussion of health care ethics. The ethos of the health sciences, particularly its experimental concepts, was profoundly influenced by the Nuremberg experience. The Nazi medical experiments conducted during World War II had their genesis in a number of historical and social trends. As early as the 1800s, German medicine and universities participated in the insidious beginnings of 20th-century anti-Semitism. A number of socio-political changes affected the physician, who, no longer an individual entrepreneur, became responsible for expressing the values of the prevailing social order. By the 1920s, emphasis on public health and preventive medicine focused on the desire to perfect the "Aryan Race" by eliminating all impurities and defects.

The horrors of Nazi medical research included such experiments on concentration camp inmates as sterilization, placing inmates in pressure chambers and forcing them to endure high-altitude atmospheres until they died, tests on the effects of weightlessness and rapid fall, and freezing experiments in ice and snow. The K-technology, or the science of killing, led the Nazis to inject inmates with lethal doses of typhus and other pathogens and to experiment on them with gas gangrene wounds, bone grafting, and direct injections of potassium and cyanide into the heart. The physicians dissected inmates alive to observe brain and heart functioning. And finally, at the height of sadism, the motivation for the macabre experiments was to collect different shapes of skulls and to retrieve human skin in order to make lampshades. The Nazi physicians' immolation of medical ethics on a massive scale proceeded unopposed by the German medical profession (Lifton, 2000). Out of this experience came the Nuremberg Code, providing valuable insights and directives for current research involving human subjects. One of this code's contributions is the precision with which it discusses the criterion of informed consent. The single most important ethical legacy of the Nuremberg experience is that it reminds us of the potential evil in human beings and serves to constantly refute the myth of inevitable progress.

For nurses, it is important to know that some of our German colleagues participated in some of these events. Specifically, nurses participated in the Nazi euthanasia measures against patients with mental and physical disabilities that killed over 100,000 patients from 1939 to 1945. According to historical records, these nurses reacted in several ways: (a) some had no conflicts of conscience, (b) others did as they were told with regret, and (c) a few refused (McFarland-Icke, 1999). We should think about what we might do under similar circumstances.

Other Documents and Individual Rights

Although not an ethical code per se, the American Hospital Association (AHA) developed a Statement on a Patient's Bill of Rights, which had implications for health care ethics. This bill, posted in all hospitals to notify patients of their rights, can be used by patients and nurses alike.

Other documents, not discussed here, also speak of the concepts of human rights and have implications for health care ethics. They are the *World Medical Association Helsinki Declaration of 1964* and the *United Nations International Covenant on Human Rights*. Since so many factors influence health and illness, these documents and selected references, addressing the larger social, economic, cultural, civil, and political rights, provide a matrix for health care ethics (Farmer, 2003; Mann, Gruskin, Grodin, & Annas, 1999; Marks, 2004; Sachs, 2005; Singer, 2004).

THE ROLE OF THE ETHICIST

To the extent that we confront and attempt to deal with ethical dilemmas in health care by ethical reasoning, we assume the role of an ethicist. One can say that each of us is an ethicist; however, there are individuals specifically trained to help health professionals with ethical dilemmas. Although these individuals may not be directly involved in the care of the patient, they can help by bringing their particular expertise to the situation. Such a person can help to conceptually structure the ethical issues involved in any ethical dilemma and provide another perspective, drawing not from a background in the health sciences but from philosophy and theology. Some health care centers now have an ethicist on the staff to assist the physicians, nurses, and others who ultimately must resolve specific ethical dilemmas and act on the decisions made. Many more facilities have ethics committees, and an urban medical center most likely will have a research ethics committee and a clinical ethics committee. Nurses serve on these committees and they need to be able to discuss aspects of ethical dilemmas. In addition, nurses in any ethical dilemma situation in a health care facility need knowledge and skill in ethics.

Although we have ethicists and ethics committees in health care settings, the fact remains that each person is a moral agent. To the extent that we develop moral sensitivity and systematic ways of reasoning through an ethical dilemma, we will do a better job at being a moral agent and a patient advocate. As nurses are even more affected by these situations in the future, they will need to recognize ethical dilemmas as such and will need to be able to think through these dilemmas so that they can participate actively in the decisions on and possible resolution of these dilemmas. It is important to be able to take an ethical stance and to be able to articulate and ethically justify it. Righteous indignation may have its place, but a thoughtful ethical stance may have more impact in the decision-making process.

Some Questions to Consider

1. What do you value?
2. What ethical position do you have on beginning-of-life and end-of-life ethical issues?
3. Do you think that you as a nurse have a duty to care for all patients even if you disagree with his or her ethics or health care decisions?
4. Have you read the Code? Recently?
5. Have you thought about the ethical issue of discrepancies in health care services?

References

American Nurses Association (ANA). (1995). *Code of Ethics for Nurses*. Silver Spring, MD: ANA.

American Nurses Association (ANA). (2004). *Nursing's social policy statement*. Washington, DC: ANA.

Bayles, M. D., & Bayles, M. (Eds.). (1990). *Contemporary utilitarianism*. Garden City, NY: Doubleday and Co.

Beauchamp, T. L., & Childress, J. F. (2001). *Principles of biomedical ethics*. New York: Oxford University Press.

Benner, P. (Ed.). (1994). *Interpretive phenomenology: Embodiment, caring, and ethics in health & Illness*. Thousand Oaks, CA: Sage Publications.

Davis, A. J., Tschudin, V., & deRaeve, L. (Eds.). (2006). *Essentials of teaching and learning in nursing ethics: Perspectives and methods*. London: Churchill Livingston.

Du Bose, E. R., Hamel, R., & O'Connell, L. J. (1994). *A matter of principles? Ferment in U.S. bioethics*. Valley Forge, PA: Trinity Press International.

Farmer, P. (2003). *Pathologies of power: Health, human rights, and the new war on the poor*. Berkeley: University of California Press.

Gilligan, C. (1982). *In a different voice*. Cambridge, MA: Harvard University Press.

Gilligan, C. (1993). *In a different voice*. Cambridge, MA: Harvard University Press.

International Council of Nurses. (2005). *Code of ethics*. Geneva: ICN.

Kohlberg, L. (1981). *The philosophy of moral development*. New York: Harper & Row.

Lifton, R. J. (2000). *The Nazi doctors: Medical killing and the psychology of genocide*. New York: Basic Books.

Mann, J. M., Gruskin, S., Grodin, M. A., & Annas, G. J. (1999). *Health and human rights*. New York: Routledge.

Marks, S. P. (Ed.). (2004). *Health and Human Rights: Basic International Documents*. Cambridge, MA: Harvard School of Public Health.

McFarland-Icke, B. (1999). *Nurses in Nazi Germany: Moral choices in history*. Princeton, NJ: Princeton University Press.

McIntyre, A. (1984). *After virtue* (2nd ed.). Notre Dame, IN: University of Notre Dame Press.

Milgram, S. (1963). Behavioral study of obedience. *Journal of Abnormal and Social Psychology, 67*, 371–378.

Noddings, N. (1984). *Caring: a feminine approach to ethics and moral education*. Berkeley: University of California Press.

Sachs, J. D. (2005). *The end of poverty*. New York: Penguin Books.

Sherman, N. (1991). *The fabric of character: Aristotle's theory of virtue*. Oxford: Clarendin Press.

Sherwin, S. (1993). *No longer patient: Feminist ethics and health care*. Philadelphia: Temple University Press.

Singer, P. (2004). *One world: The ethics of globalization*. New Haven, CT: Yale University Press.

Thomson, T. T. (1990). *The realm of rights*. Cambridge, MA: Harvard University Press.

CHAPTER 2

Selected Ethical Approaches: Theories and Concepts

Ethical issues and questions confronted nurses even before the founding of modern nursing by Florence Nightingale. Yet, the late 20th and early 21st centuries bring new and daunting challenges. While intensive care units (ICUs) are now commonplace, we forget that they arose in the 1960s with the development of new diagnostic and treatment technologies. End-of-life ethical issues came to the fore, particularly in discussions of unwarranted or unwanted treatment, "slow codes," do-not-resuscitate (DNR) orders, and "futility." At the same time, concerns for the cost of care and access to it became and remain acute. Diagnosis-related groups (DRGs), health maintenance organizations (HMOs), managed care, and other measures of cost containment or cost reduction, such as downsizing, gatekeeping, and changing patient–nurse ratios, affected and continue to affect the environment in which nursing is practiced. Population changes too raise ethical issues. The aging of our society and widespread obesity, even among the youth and children, raise new ethical challenges for health and preventive care. The increased number of non-Western European immigrants, as well as a heightened recognition of the plight of our own indigenous peoples, challenges our cultural sensitivity and intercultural moral aptitude. For those who had a grandmother who was a nurse—these are not your grandmother's ethical problems!

Nurses make judgments every day that affect human lives at critical junctures. Many of these situations involve relationships and decisions in which there are conflicts of values, priorities, duties, and ideals related to what is "good" or "right" for individuals, families, communities, and society as well as for the nursing profession itself. Nurses encounter situations in their daily work in which ethical questions and concerns require an order of judgment different from that of clinical judgments. Decision making regarding end-of-life issues of patients and the allocation of professional nursing expertise in downsizing hospitals, including ICUs, push nurses to respond to the ethical aspects of practice and answers are not easy.

Gut-level feelings or past practice is substantially less than adequate as a basis for responding to the complex moral conflicts or dilemmas that confront nurses today. The stakes are too high. A more systematic and consistent way of approaching ethical aspects of practice is required in responding to difficult decisions and choices in which ethical principles and values such as respect for persons and avoiding harm often conflict. These are not bedside issues alone. The issues also rise to the level of organizational policy and health care or public policy making. An appropriate ethical approach requires the use of a reasoned process in which explicit attention is paid to the ethical aspects of nursing practice.

The content of ethical decisions in nursing and health care is changing as the field of bioethics is evolving from a primary focus on philosophical theories that emphasize formal principles to a broader array of ethical approaches. This chapter is a brief introduction to selected ethical theories and concepts that can be considered in responding to patient care situations where what is right or good is unclear or where there is a conflict between nursing duties and obligations. Ethical theories and approaches presented here are virtue ethics with a focus on individual character, utilitarianism, deontology that focuses on principles, and caring as one aspect of feminist ethics with a focus on relationships and responsibilities.

The concerns of ethics have to do with examining the moral basis for our judgments and actions, our duties and obligations. Moral philosophers and theologians across the centuries have attempted to answer questions of ethics such as, "How can we know what is right?" This question falls in the division of ethics called *metaethics*. Two major concerns are addressed by the division of ethics called *normative ethics*: What is right *to do*? What is morally good for a person *to be* or cherish? Nurses and other health professionals are primarily concerned with normative ethics. Applied normative ethics, sometimes called clinical ethics or practice ethics, is derived from normative ethics. Normative ethics attempts to justify one form of behavior over another and to determine the characteristics of an action that make it right, ultimately for the purpose of identifying and carrying out one's professional duties and obligations when they are unclear. Nurses often find themselves in ethical dilemmas that require choices between alternative courses of action that seem equally unattractive. Choices must be made that have significant implications for patient well-being and often the well-being of others. Applied normative ethics is also concerned about the moral attributes of the nurse, that is, the "morally good nurse," as moral character is essential to moral action. A decision-making framework, along with standards of nursing practice and codes of professional ethics, is helpful in reflecting on moral decision making regarding actions to take, as well as the moral character of the nurse. The framework presented here contains elements that are familiar from the nursing process and adds ethical considerations in a more systematic way. These ethical elements will be discussed in more detail later in this chapter as ethical theories and concepts.

ELEMENTS OF A DECISION-MAKING FRAMEWORK

The ability to provide an ethically supportable rationale for decisions and actions is foundational to professional practice and to the integrity of practitioners in all arenas and forms of nursing practice. The reflective decision-making framework presented here can be used in responding to the ethical questions posed by the case studies found at the end of each of the chapters. The first task is to identify whether a situation presents an ethical dilemma or problem recognizing that the nurse–patient relationship always has ethical dimensions whether problematic or not. Fundamentally, an ethical dilemma involves a conflict of moral duties or a conflict of moral values. The first step in the decisional process is to identify whether or not a conflict of moral duties or values exists.

Once a situation is identified that constitutes an ethical problem, consideration of the following elements assists with the discussion, analysis, and development of ethically supportable decisions. These elements can be adapted for use at the policy development or evaluation level, as well as used for ethical problems related to individual patient care decisions. They include the following:

1. Review of the overall situation to identify what is going on
2. Identification of the significant facts about the patient (client), including medical, social history, decision-making capacity, existence of an advance directive for treatment
3. Identification of the parties or stakeholders involved in the situation or affected by the decision(s) that is made
4. Identification of morally relevant legal data
5. Identification of specific conflicts of ethical principles or values
6. Identification of possible choices, their intent, and probable consequences for the welfare of the patient(s) as the primary concern
7. Identification of practical constraints (e.g., legal, organizational, political, and economic) and facilitators (e.g., an ethics committee or clinical ethicist)
8. Make recommendations for action that are determined to be ethically supportable recognizing that the possible choices often have both positive and negative consequences
9. Take action if you are the decision maker and implementer of the decision(s) made
10. Review and evaluate the situation after action is taken in order to determine what was learned that will help in resolution of similar situations in patient care and related policy development

This process indicates that the methods of thinking in science and ethics are not mutually exclusive. One goes through a similar process of discernment in asking questions about the world of nature, on the one hand, and the world of ethics and values, on the other hand. The database is different as are the variables considered, but both are reflective processes that can be learned.

Different ethical theories provide different emphases and ways of reasoning in an ethically substantive way. Ethics can often assist in determining the boundaries of a morally acceptable action and, within those boundaries, may identify more than one morally supportable approach. The range of morally difficult situations that nurses face is extensive and includes end-of-life decisions, allocation of nursing resources, use of children as human subjects in research, concern for the impaired practice of a colleague, and access to nursing and health care nationally. Because these situations are often frustrating and painful to deal with, a spirit of compassion and caring is necessary in making the difficult choices involved whether at the bedside or in policy making. The first theoretical approach to be discussed focuses on the character or virtues of the decision makers.

FOCUS ON VIRTUE AND CHARACTER

For the past three decades, the bioethics literature has focused much more heavily on the process and content of ethical decision making with less attention given to questions of moral character. Now, there is a resurgence of concern for the character of decision makers, a traditional concern of ethics and moral philosophy, as well as the content and process of decision making (MacIntyre, 1966). Issues of character are significant to professional practice broadly and more narrowly to development of responses to ethical issues in patient care and policy making (Begley, 2005). It can be argued that the character and integrity of nurses as individual moral agents determine, or at the very least influence, whether ethical problems are identified and how responses are developed to such problems in patient care and policy arenas. *Virtues* are the elements of desirable moral character and refer to particular dispositions or learned "habits-of-being," such as integrity, trustworthiness, respectfulness, honesty, and kindness. They are evidenced by our behavior and enable nurses to live out their ethical obligations such as truthfulness or respect for individuals as self-determining and as interconnected members of the human community. While the major provisions of the ANA *Code of Ethics for Nurses* (2001) allude to virtues that are necessary for ethical nursing practice, such as competence, the *Code* acknowledges that it cannot assure the character of each individual nurse (American Nurses Association, 2001).

Philosopher of clinical ethics James Drane describes what he calls a virtue approach to bioethics, in which he argues that considerations of character and virtue, often considered to be too subjective, do have a place in today's professional health care ethics in order to enrich a field currently characterized by a focus on right decisions and acts based on consideration of more abstract ethical principles (Drane, 1994). Descriptions of moral character and moral character traits portray a way of *being* instead of a way of acting. These traits are learned or habituated and are not to be confused with personality traits. When positive or good, they are called *virtues*; when negative or evil, they are called *vices*. The nurse who responds to a difficult patient care situation with respect, patience, and an attitude of care is described as a "good" nurse or a "good" person in a moral sense, whereas the nurse who responds to the same situation with impatience and disrespect for a patient and family would not be viewed in the same way. Moral conduct flows from what we are as moral agents; what we are as moral agents influences both professional and personal behavior. These two elements, nurses' ways of being and of acting, are integral to the quality and integrity of nursing practice and patient care. One's character is a source as well as the product of one's value commitments and actions. In turn, one's character and behaviors are also influenced by one's social (work) environment. This provides an argument for attention to organizational ethics in health care systems, where existing power differentials between and among nurses, physicians, patients, and payers and differing goals for health care must be considered as part of the milieu of nursing practice and decision making.

FOCUS ON PRINCIPLES

Two ethical theories or approaches that have been emphasized in bioethics over the past few decades are deontology (from Greek *deon*, meaning duty), specifically Immanuel Kant's form of deontology, and John Stuart Mill's Utilitarianism. These theories have been dominant in bioethics but have become less so in recent years (Clouser & Gert, 1990).

Kantian formalism determines an action to be right or wrong based upon the conformity of that action to a "form," that is, a rule or moral principle (Kant, 1964). Utilitarianism determines an action to be right or wrong based upon the consequences of the action as measured against a specific desired end, such as social *utility* (Mill, 2002). Rule-based Utilitarianism employs rules, as do deontological theories, but for different reasons: specifically that conformity to a moral rule will in general produce the desired consequences (Rosen, 2003). These theories provide different ethical arguments and perspectives from which to consider decisions in troubling patient care or policy development situations. They may, nonetheless, arrive at the same conclusion via different means/theories. Both are discussed here in more detail than the other theoretical approaches because they continue to dominate the thinking of clinical ethics and health policy development implicitly and explicitly in our society.

Ethical Theory Based on Multiple Principles

The most common deontological theory that is used is that of Kantian Formalism, or Kantianism, attributed to the 18th-century moral philosopher Immanuel Kant. This theory focuses on specifying moral duties through the use of principles. Whether an act is right or wrong depends on more than an individual's preferences, pleasure, or the consequences of the proposed action. Rightness or wrongness of an action depends on the inherent moral significance of the action, that is, its conformity to a moral rule, for example the rule of promise-keeping. These principles are seen as universal, that is, all persons including myself ought to affirm them in our moral decisions and actions. They are also universal in the sense that they are always to be applied. That is, when one makes a moral judgment in a given situation, one will make the same judgment in any similar situation regardless of time, place, or persons involved. If one judges X to be right or good in this situation, then one must judge that X is right or good in any similar situation (Frankena, 1973). In Kantianism or rule deontology, problems arise when two principles conflict. Two questions arise here: How are we to know what the moral principles are? How are we to arbitrate a conflict between two principles?

Kant had a rule for moral rule making, called the *categorical imperative*. He had three formulations of this one rule, and he claimed that the three formulations were identical, that is, that they were identical as restatements and were not different rules. The best-known formulation is "act only on that maxim which you can at the same time will to be a universal law" (Frankena, 1973, p. 30). This formulation emphasizes the question, "Would we want all persons to observe this principle or rule under similar circumstances?" Kant's second formulation of the categorical imperative states "always use humans, whether in your own person or that of another, never as a means only, but always at one and the same time as an end also." What is meant by this? We cannot use patients, or nursing students, or human subjects, or any others, as ends to *our* own means only—these persons must always be an end in themselves as well. This represents an ethical challenge to nurse researchers who use hospital patients or nursing home residents primarily or nursing students as means to nursing research goals. Kant maintained that principles that derive from the categorical imperative are unconditional, morally necessary, and a duty for all under any similar circumstances (Kant, 1965).

What are the principles and rules that arise for the categorical imperative? They include respecting the autonomy of others, not harming others, doing good for others, justice, gratitude, reparations, promise keeping, truth telling, and more. In the more specific language of ethics, *principles* tend to be broader and more overarching, while *rules* tend to be derived from principles (Beauchamp & Childress, 2001). Nevertheless, the terms *principles* and *rules* tend to be used interchangeably. These rules and principles provide a basis for analysis and further provide guidance in specifying our ethical duties. In instances of moral dilemmas, we then ought to engage in moral actions that fulfill those duties.

Sometimes, however, we find that two rules or principles conflict, that is, when we have two duties that arise that are mutually exclusive and conflicting. Other times, we are confronted with a situation that appears to be an "exception to the rule." In dealing with these problems, W. D. Ross distinguished between what he called *actual duties* and *prima facie duties. Prima facie* is Latin for "on its first appearance," or as we might say, "at first glance." *Prima facie* obligations are duties that we must always try to meet—for example, fidelity, gratitude, beneficence (doing good), nonmaleficence (not inflicting harm), and justice (Ross, 2002). But sometimes these duties conflict with another duty. For example, a nurse has promised a patient to return very shortly with a pain medication and to assist with ambulation. Then, another patient has a cardiac arrest and the nurse is caught up in the "code blue" and does not keep her or his promise to return with pain medication and to assist with post-op ambulation. While meeting one duty to do good for the patient experiencing cardiac arrest, the nurse is violating the duty to keep a promise. Ross maintains that prima facie duties are conditional, that is, that they are binding *unless* superseded by another duty. While there is no hierarchy of duties for Ross, situations will make one duty more incumbent than another, that is, one duty is more important than the other in this situation. This more incumbent duty is what Ross calls an *actual duty* and it takes priority over *prima facie* or *conditional* duties. In this situation, trying to save a life is a more important duty than returning with a pain medication; that is, beneficence (doing good) is more important in this instance than is promise keeping (Ross, 1970).

In the 1970s, an important work, *Principles of Biomedical Ethics*, was published by Beauchamp and Childress. It subsequently became a standard in bioethics and remains an important work today in its fifth edition (Beauchamp & Childress, 2001). Beauchamp and Childress identify four principles from which, they maintain, all other rules are derived. The four principles are *respect for autonomy, nonmaleficence, beneficence,* and *justice.* The first three named are "bedside principles" in that they constantly arise in dilemmas in clinical practice, as well as in other arenas of nursing practice. The three principles also tend to be the language of institutional ethics committees. Justice, as a principle, arises as a consideration of larger groups, such as institutions, regional agencies, or national policy. For the moment, considerations of the principle of justice will be set aside.

The principle of *respect for persons* is broader than a principle that speaks to respect for individual autonomy and self-determination. In addition to respect for individual autonomy, it also recognizes that individuals are interrelated and interconnected members of the human community. The broader principle, emphasized in nursing, recognizes that many of the decisions we make as individuals affect others, directly or indirectly, and it rejects an extreme ethic of individualism with an overemphasis on individual rights. Respect for persons requires that each individual be treated as unique and as of equal worth to every other individual.

Respect for autonomy requires specific justification for interference with an individual's own purposes, privacy, or behavior (Jonsen & Butler, 1975). This principle rules out *paternalism* on the part of health professionals toward patients with decision-making capacity. It further requires that patients' own goals and values be taken into account in decisions about care and treatment if patients are unable to make their own decisions. The larger principle of respect for persons as individuals and as interconnected community members requires consideration of duties and obligations to others—all others—as well as to one's self. Commitment to the principle of respect for persons affects whether and how ethically troubling situations are dealt with on a patient care unit and influences all of the relationships on that unit. It can be used as one ethical benchmark for evaluating nurse–patient interactions and organizational policies. In addition to considering the patient as an autonomous individual, nurses would think about patients as members of families and communities when considering nurses' obligations as patient advocates. Morally, nurses may not just follow the physician's orders, when those orders ride roughshod over patient choices, or when they ignore important patient attributes, or when they have untoward consequences for others. The same is true of "institutional policy." Neither physician order nor institutional policy dissolves a nurse's moral duties.

Respect for persons as a general guide to decisions and actions has consequences for individual patients, health professionals, and health care organizations. Decision making may become a more time-consuming process when one has to attend to multiple stakeholders. There will always be emergency situations in which health professionals will make decisions without immediate patient input—for example, in emergencies, beneficence (preserving life) generally trumps respect for autonomy (getting consent). Yet, the principle of respect for autonomy places the burden on the nurse to provide adequate moral justification for failing to secure patient participation in a health care decision. Respect for autonomy also requires of nurses that they not override an informed and consenting patient decision because they think it a bad decision. This is called *paternalism* (Gert, Culver, & Clauser, 2006). If respect for autonomy is to have any meaning, we must respect patient's decisions when they make decisions we agree with as well as when we do not. Organizational structures can also be subject to analysis using the principles of respect for persons and respect for autonomy. Does the organization value nurses as it values physicians? Are nurses given a say in patient care decisions?

The principle of nonmaleficence is a *negative duty*, that is a duty in which one *refrains* from acting. Beneficence is a *positive duty* in that it requires that one take an action. Sometimes the principle of nonmaleficence (the noninfliction of harm) is combined with the principle of beneficence (preventing harm, removing harmful conditions, and positively benefitting another), in which case it is called the principle of beneficence. While it is easy to separate the nonmaleficence from beneficence for the purposes of discussion, in nursing practice their separation is not so divisible. The combined principle of beneficence provides a continuum of action from the noninfliction of harm to positively benefitting another. (Beauchamp & Childress, 2001).

According to moral philosopher William Frankena, both nonmaleficence and beneficence are obligations that one must try to fulfill, though at times they may conflict
(Frankena, 1973, p. 47). One example is infant immunizations. Overall, they inflict
some degree of short-term pain but have long-term health benefits. Or, one might
consider a surgical procedure that inflicts immediate harm and risk of harm (the
incision, opening the peritoneum, administration of anesthesia, and so forth) in order
to promote a positive outcome such as removing an inflamed appendix. Frankena
points out that these principles apply to everyone and thus are universal (Frankena,
1973, p. 24). Philosophers Beauchamp and Childress take the position that nonmaleficence also requires moral agents such as nurses to be reflective about their
decisions and actions and to follow professional standards of care as moral obligations (Beauchamp & Childress, 2001).

The beneficence principle requires the provision of benefits and a balancing of
harms and benefits as well (Beauchamp & Childress, 2001, pp. 292–293). Benefits
related to health are considered to have positive value that promotes health or welfare,
such as the prevention of illness or premature death. Costs, while usually thought of in
financial terms, can be anything that detracts from human health and welfare, such as
physical or psychological pain. Since some costs are predictive (i.e., not immediate),
they are often referred to as risks. Risks refer to potential future harms. Weighing of
risks and benefits in patient care decision making, human subjects research, or policy
development can be considered as part of the thoughtful and careful action required
by the principle of beneficence. Risks must be assessed and balanced against potential
benefits to the patient, from the perspective of the patient or persons affected, not
from the perspective of the nurse. That is, the patient's value structure prevails in the
determination of benefit, cost, and risk (ANA, 2001). By their nature, risks and benefits
have an element of uncertainty in their calculation.

This same balancing must also be done at the state and national level of health
policy. Examples include balancing of the trade-offs required in development of
national organ transplant policies when there is a scarcity of available organs for the
people who could potentially benefit. Or, consider national disagreements over the use
of costly technologies for the prolongation of life in elderly patients when a greater
number of younger patients might benefit if treatments were withheld from the elderly
and resources conserved for society (Callahan, 2003).

While the principles of respect for persons, respect for autonomy, nonmaleficence, and beneficence have clear application at the microlevel, the principle of
justice is more commonly used in midlevel or macrolevel considerations. The range of
considerations under the principle of justice are broad and would include such things
as determining the number and kind of nursing home beds that will be authorized and
licensed in a given geographic area; how vaccines for flu and other diseases will be
distributed and who will get them first; and who should get what levels of nursing care
in a hospital that is downsizing nursing staff.

Ideas about justice are basic to the structure of a society and to social structures for
delivery of nursing and health care. There are many ways of talking about justice in our
pluralistic society. We do not currently have a social consensus as to what exactly constitutes justice, although it is recognized that most people have a sense of justice. Most of
us would probably agree on what constitutes injustice—lack of access to needed health
care for the working poor, for example (MacIntyre, 1989).

Distributive justice is one of several types of justice and has to do with the distribution or allocation of goods and evils, or burdens and benefits, in society. Sometimes, there are conditions of scarcity that complicate the consideration. Rationing is also a concern of the principle of justice. Distributive justice is a particularly relevant form of justice for discussions of health care access, cost, and allocation.

How are resources (e.g., public education, fire fighting) and the burdens (e.g., taxation) of those resources to be allocated? Are resources to be allocated equally? Are there differences between individuals or groups that would warrant unequal distribution? If so, what might be a morally relevant difference, as opposed to a prejudicial difference? How might these considerations affect the allocation of health care resources?

There are several ideas as to what might serve as justification for different distribution of benefits and costs of health care to individuals or groups. These ideas include individual need, individual effort, merit (achievement), ability to pay, societal contribution, social contract, and that there are no morally relevant differences. Different bases for distribution are used in different contexts. For example, welfare payments are distributed on the basis of need, while jobs and promotions are usually distributed on the basis of individual achievement or merit (MacIntyre, 1989, p. 331). Grades in schools are customarily based on merit, though they may include a small "reward" figured in based on the effort the student makes. But what bases should apply to the distribution of the burdens and benefits of health care: effort to be healty? age? sex? weight? nonsmoker? bad health habits? As alluded to above, age has been suggested as a criterion for the distribution of benefits of health care, specifically high-tech care at the end of life (Callahan, 2008).

Individual need is commonly invoked in nursing documents such as the ANA *Code of Ethics for Nurses* to justify the distribution of the benefits of nursing and health care (ANA, 2001). Health maintenance organizations and other types of managed care organizations often use the language of "medical necessity" (i.e., medical *need*) to determine plan benefits. One issue in using the concept of need as a basis for just distribution is who defines needs vis-à-vis demands, wants, or fundamental needs. A *fundamental need* refers to something such as emergency care for chest pain, which indicates that a person is immanently at risk of harm if care is not obtained.

The work of philosopher John Rawls on justice as fairness and justice as the foundation of social structures provides another way of looking at a more just distribution of social goods, such as work, income, and self-respect (Rawls, 1971). According to Rawls, the principles of justice have to do with distribution of what he called primary goods: income, wealth, liberty, opportunity, and the bases of self-respect. His theory offers another perspective from which to view ethical decision making and the basis for moral decisions in health care, particularly at the level of national policy, even though Rawls made no claim that his theory could be applied directly to economic or social issues in contemporary society. His ideas about justice are based on a rethinking of the social contract theory of obligation in the Kantian tradition. The heart of the theory is the notion of the "original position," in which people come together to negotiate the principles of justice by which all are bound to live. A part of the "original position" construct is that the individuals are deciding for others but do not know who the others are and do not even know their own situation in life; they are behind a *veil of ignorance*, and those others for whom they are deciding could be a loved one or a stranger. The negotiators are rational, intelligent people who wish to pursue their own life plans in a more just society (Rawls, 1971, pp. 17–22, 62, 136–147). The purpose of the veil of ignorance is to remove from the negotiations any possibility of individuals seeking to satisfy their own interests at the expense of others, or the interests of their friends over others. This is the situation referred to as the "original position." The negotiators must favor only those principles that advance everyone's best interests. Any of the negotiators might turn out to be one of the least fortunate or less advantaged individuals in a given community (Rawls, 1971, pp. 136–142). In the end, the negotiators must arrive at what Rawls called "justice as fairness," because they negotiate behind the veil of ignorance to form the basic principles of a just society (Rawls, 1971, p. 302).

Rawls' concept of justice as fairness is articulated in two basic principles of justice: (a) each person is to have an equal right to the most extensive system of liberty for all; and (b) social and economic inequalities are to be arranged so that they are to the greatest benefit of the least fortunate and are attached to offices and positions open to everyone under conditions of equality of opportunity (Rawls, 1999). The first principle, maximizing liberty for all, has absolute priority over the second if and when the two principles conflict. Rawls also discussed five criteria for judging the "rightness" of any ethical principle: (a) *universality* (i.e., the same principles must hold for everyone in similar situations), (b) *generality* (i.e., the principles must not refer to specific people or situations, such as my mother or your marriage), (c) *publicity* (i.e., the criteria must be known and recognized by all involved), (d) *ordering* (i.e., the criteria must somehow order conflicting claims without resorting to force), and (e) *finality* (i.e., the criteria may override the demands of law and custom) (Rawls, 1999, pp. 131–135). Nurses could use these criteria to examine their own moral principles used in decision making, those proposed by other health professionals or those assumed in a policy for health care delivery to those who are uninsured (Rawls, 1999, pp. 131–135).

In Rawls' theory of justice as fairness, inequalities are allowed only to improve the condition of the least fortunate or most vulnerable—for example, children, the frail elderly, and the poor. The least advantaged then are in the normative position in society, that is their situation is determinative of how inequalities are to be addressed. Basic rights and obligations proceed from the notion of fairness for these disadvantaged groups. Justice as fairness to the least advantaged becomes a categorical imperative in the Kantian tradition. Rawls has provided us with a way to look at moral problems in society generally and to critically examine the distribution of finite economic and nursing resources in health care. Meeting health care needs in our society amid changes such as development and use of new health care technologies and rationing of health care for the poor and uninsured require attention to issues of distributive justice, in which Rawls' understanding of justice as fairness is useful and consistent with the value structure of the nursing profession and its concern for vulnerable populations. Using income inequalities and ability to pay as screening devices for access to health care is ethically unjustifiable under this view of justice and is inconsistent with the ANA *Code of Ethics for Nurses* (2001).

Briefly returning to Kantian ethical theory, it does not help us with the resolution of conflict between moral principles as Ross attempts to do with the ideas of actual and prima facie duties. When one tries to apply the Kantian theory of obligation, it is difficult to separate the idea of duty and obligations from ends, purposes, wants, and needs in any given situation. For example, if the goal is to return the institutionalized developmentally disabled to the community, what happens to the specific needs of a particular developmentally disabled adult who may not be able to live outside an institution and has no family? What is a health provider's obligation or what type of health policy is required to respond to this and similar issues?

In summary, the deontological or Kantian theoretical approach focuses on the moral significance of the values of the moral agent or decision maker and on duties and obligations guided by specific rules and principles without regard to consequences. Consequences are not unimportant; they just do not serve as the criterion for determining whether an action is right or wrong. This position does not help nurses as moral agents resolve situations in which duties and obligations conflict and choices must be made. It does not resolve the dilemma for the nurse who decides to follow the rule that one should always tell the truth and realizes that the truth will undoubtedly hurt a particular patient in a given situation, creating a conflict between the rule of telling the truth and the principle of doing no harm. Kantian ethics, however limited, does provide us with one way to consider what counts from an ethical perspective in a patient care situation where there is disagreement about medical interventions or in health policy development that has consequences for the most vulnerable. From an ethical perspective, we cannot ignore considerations of respect for persons, avoiding harm, beneficence, and justice in healthcare decision making.

Ethical Theory Based on a Single Principle

The theory of utility or *utilitarianism* is one form of consequentialistic theory using the single principle of utility. It focuses on consequences of decisions and actions and defines "good" as happiness or pleasure and "the right" as maximizing the greatest good and least amount of harm for the greatest number of persons. Whatever maximizes utility as happiness or pleasure is to be pursued. This position assumes that one can weigh and measure harms and benefits and arrive at the greatest possible balance of good over evil for most people.

Jeremy Bentham and John Stuart Mill have presented the major historical arguments for the position of utility as a standard against which the rightness and wrongness of actions are to be compared (Mill, 2002). This position, sometimes known as calculus morality, calculates the effects of all alternative actions on the general welfare of present and future generations in a given situation. Some moral philosophers distinguish between rule- and act-utilitarianism. One seeks to determine acts and rules having the greatest utility in a broad sense of usefulness, pleasure, and happiness. The agent looks at actions and rules in terms of what the consequences would be for the general welfare if everyone acted similarly in a given situation (Frankena, 1973, pp. 39–41). What if every hospital decided to perform heart transplants and to close its emergency room? What would be the consequences for a population group that uses an emergency room as its only source for primary care?

One is immediately faced with the problem of aggregation in this theory focused on consequences. Does this theory involve aggregation of total happiness for a few or average happiness for all? A crucial question is whether or not what one does in a particular situation contributes to the greatest general good or the least amount of harm for everyone. But how can everyone's welfare really be considered in a large, pluralistic society of millions of people or even in large hospitals or nursing homes? Critics bring up several other problems. They accuse the utilitarian of ignoring the personal nature of good as exemplified in truth telling and promise keeping. All actions need not be considered in light of the overall general welfare. Each individual does count as one of the aggregate in this theory but one could end up in a minority group rather than the majority when consequences are identified.

A utilitarian approach is often invoked in making decisions about the funding and delivery of health care. This is in direct conflict with the medical ethic in which everything possible is done for the individual patient. Also, some individuals or groups may accept benefits without making any sacrifices, raising the "free rider" issue. Questions of justice and fairness, and rights and responsibilities, are not adequately addressed by utilitarianism. Utility is not the only criterion in making moral judgments. If one does add the notion of distributing the good as widely as possible through society, one adds the principle of justice to the principle of utility for making ethical judgments. This is no longer pure utilitarianism. From this point of view, utility by itself cannot be the only basic standard or first principle of right and wrong and requires consideration of at least two principles (utility *and* justice) in decision making that count from an ethical perspective (Frankena, 1973, pp. 42–43).

To summarize, deontological and utilitarian traditions offer different perspectives from which moral judgments might be made and ethical problems assessed using a principled approach of multiple principles or a single principle. Each position has strengths and limitations when considered in the context of specific ethical dilemmas in nursing and health care delivery, where readymade responses do not exist and moral discernment is required. Kantian theory could be viewed as more sympathetic with virtue or character ethics given its consideration of persons as moral agents. Even in a theory of utility, it is hard to totally ignore the moral character of decision makers who do the aggregating and decide ultimately what counts as morally significant consequences such as in development of institutional or public policy that involves financing and delivery of health care.

FOCUS ON CARING

Today's philosophers and bioethicists offer other theoretical positions from which to look at ethical dilemmas and problems in a richer and more comprehensive way than the use of abstract principles alone, such as theoretical approaches focused on character and caring as points of departure for ethical discussion and decision making. Even in these approaches, one can discern hints of principles although the substantive content of these theories is not couched in the language of abstract principles. These perspectives also have their strengths and limitations and demonstrate that we do not have a single overarching ethical theory to explain how we identify the rightness or wrongness of decisions and actions. An ethic of caring with a focus on relationships and responsibility will be discussed here as one aspect of the broader field of feminist ethics. According to Christine Gudorf, a professor of religious studies, feminist approaches to biomedical ethics in the United States have developed primarily from women's lived experience of alienation within the health care system rather than as a critique of ethical principlism as ethics based on abstract principles (Gudorf, 1994).

The idea of an ethic of caring is appealing to nurses who consider the foundations of their practice to be about caring—caring for people, for the environment, for society, and for the profession. Contemporary nurse philosopher Sarah Fry proposes caring as a fundamental value for the development of a theory of nursing ethics (Fry, 1989). Caring, viewed as a value "is of central importance in the nurse–patient relationship," is considered as "a pre-condition for the care of specific entities, whether things, others, or oneself," and "is identified with moral and social ideals" (Fry, 1989, p. 15). Care for particular others is a core notion in an ethic of care according to philosopher Nel Noddings (Noddings, 2003). This core notion is evident in the ANA *Code of Ethics* (2001), which emphasizes respectful care of individuals as a major tenet. In an ethic of care, decision making focuses on identifying decisions and actions that promote and maintain relationships as an individual responsibility. Patients are viewed as unique individuals within networks of relationships rather than as isolated bodies or members of a population group—more akin to the ethical principle of respect for persons as interrelated members of the human community rather than an emphasis on individual autonomy. In health care settings, persons significant to the patient ought to be included in discussions and decision making under this idea of caring.

In her critique of ethical theories based on abstract principles, philosopher Susan Sherwin reminds us that Western philosophical ethics, focused on more abstract principles, was developed primarily by men who considered women to be morally inferior to themselves (Sherwin, 1992). Moral thought was considered to need a level of generality which most women were not thought to be capable of. Psychologist Carol Gilligan's research in the late 1970s and early 1980s found that women bring a different focus to deliberating about moral questions (Gilligan, 1993). The focus is on care and responsibility in relationships rather than on the application of abstract principles such as respect for individual autonomy and justice. Ideally, according to Gilligan, moral agents, including health professionals, are concerned about both relationships and ethical principles as they make decisions and establish practices that are morally sensitive and justifiable (Gilligan, 1993).

From a societal and historical perspective, caring has usually been the responsibility of women in the home and workplace. That continues to be the case when one looks at the majority of caregivers for children, the chronically ill, the elderly, or people with AIDS. Sherwin makes the point that "most women experience the world as a complex web of interdependent relationships where responsible caring for others is implicit in their moral lives," implying that this reality must be accounted for in theoretical and applied ethics (Gilligan, 1993, p. 47). Caring as a concept or theory for discerning right responses in ethically troubling situations is not yet well developed and requires further philosophical, scientific, and historical work (Morse, Bottorff, Neander, & Solberg, 1991). This limitation is significant for nurses and the nursing profession to consider, if caring is to serve as the basis for its professional ethic as some would propose (Davis & Fowler, 2006).

Caring focused on individuals and relationships is one aspect of feminist ethics. There is a range of "critical theories" in ethics, such as post-colonial theory, that is concerned about relationships of power, who is at the center, and who is at the margins, and whose voice is heard or not heard. Feminist ethics finds another equally compelling dimension of ethics in the analysis of oppression and dominance wherever they occur in relationships and social institutions. Oppression and dominance are found in relationships within health care organizations and in the ways that these organizations are structured to meet their goals. Power differentials between and among nurses, physicians, patients, administrators, and payors illustrate some of the relationship inequalities that exist in most health care organizations. A concern of

Sherwin's is that some women may be so focused on caring for others and meeting their needs that they may even protect those who oppress them. In doing so, they maintain a morally problematic status quo (Sherwin, 1992). The ability to care, respect for persons, avoiding harm, and justice as fairness may all be at stake or in conflict in such morally troubling situations. This aspect of feminist ethics, as a critique of caring serving as a sole basis for ethics, is important for nursing.

Nursing remains predominately a female profession and should explore both dimensions of feminist ethics in the development of decision-making processes and policies in patient care situations and organizational arrangements. Additional features of feminist ethics include incorporation of efforts to develop new nonoppressive relationships and structures for political and social interaction and to incorporate more socially oriented principles such as mutuality, community, empathy, solidarity, and integrity. Gudorf maintains that we do not need to reject principles per se but need to connect the use of principles with an examination of the concrete situation of those who are most vulnerable or most at risk (Gudorf, 1994, pp. 168, 171). All of these aspects and values are significant to the development of an adequate nursing ethics for the new millennium. An ethical benchmark for relationships in and structures of health care financing and delivery is how they contribute to the humanity of all the participants in our health care systems—systems in which no one is excluded from decisions and deliberations based on personal characteristics such as gender, race, or socioeconomic status. Such an approach links nursing's focus on respectful care of individual clients and Florence Nightingale's focus on nursing's obligation to create healing environments with the foundational values of public health—promotion of the common good and assuring conditions in which people can be healthy (Nightingale, 2007). This is a very different model and starting point for considering what is "right" in an ethically problematic situation than a focus on individualism and individual rights—still a dominant value perspective in U.S. society and in medical care.

ETHICAL THEORIES AND CONCEPTS IN NURSING PRACTICE

This limited discussion of theoretical approaches and concepts is not meant to provide the reader with a complete review of ethical theories, which requires a book in itself. Neither is this discussion intended to provide "formulas" for the resolution of ethical dilemmas in practice. It does serve to provide examples of the ethical elements to be considered in using the decision-making framework presented at the beginning of the chapter. In complex decision-making situations where ethical concerns predominate, ethical theories and concepts may well conflict or be inadequate for the task at hand. Yet, one may find any of these theories, concepts, or a combination of them, represented in health care deliberations about ethical problems whether or not they are made explicit. Ethical problems and concerns are found on a spectrum that ranges from morally troubling individual nurse–patient, nurse–nurse, or nurse–physician relationships to policy making for health plan benefits or for population-based health programs.

Nurses, both as individuals and in collaboration with others, may consider these theories and concepts as they deliberate and develop responses to questions of what is morally right to do in situations of moral conflict. A key objective is that decisions be made in a more thoughtful, reasoned way, incorporating explicit attention to ethical considerations. Part of learning skills to initiate and participate in such decision-making processes and organizational structures is to gain familiarity with ethical theories and concepts in the search to determine one's professional obligations when there are no ready-made answers, confidence in developing an ethically supportable rationale for one's decisions, and the capability to understand why and what ethical and value disagreements occur in a given situation.

Nurses might also take a look at recurrent ethical dilemmas in their practice, whether in service, education, research, or administration, and take action to modify or prevent them from happening in a spirit of preventive ethics. Some recurring dilemmas could be prevented from occurring at the primary level of prevention through listening, careful assessment, and education in dealing with hard choices about care and treatment in patient, colleague, and family relationships. Such ethical issues as informed consent and decision making, humane care of the terminally ill and dying, and experimentation with human subjects better lend themselves to a preventive approach when considered in noncrisis settings such as in planned ethics rounds, in the work of institutional ethics committees, and in the deliberations of review boards for protection of human subjects in clinical research. Such activities are an expression of the concept of fidelity, that is, faithfulness and commitment to patients as foundational to the nurse–patient relationship and to the integrity of the nursing profession as an essential service in society.

References

American Nurses Association (ANA). (2001). *Code of ethics for nurses with interpretive statements*. Silver Spring, MD: ANA.

Beauchamp, T. L., & Childress, J. F. (2001). *Principles of biomedical ethics* (5th ed.). New York: Oxford.

Begley, A. M. (2005, November). Practising virtue: A challenge to the view that a virtue centred approach to ethics lacks practical content. *Nursing Ethics, 12*(6), 622–637.

Callahan, D. (2003). *What kind of life: The limits of medical progress*. Georgetown, Washington, DC: Georgetown University Press.

Callahan, D. (2008, June). *American medical association journal of ethics: Virtual mentor, 10*(6), 404–410.

Clouser, K. D., & Gert, B. (1990). A critique of principlism. *The Journal of Medicine and Philosophy, 15*(2), 219–236.

Davis, A., & Fowler, M. (2006). Caring and caring ethics depicted in selected literature: What we know and what we need to ask. In A. Davis, V. Tschudin, & L. deRaeve (Eds.), *Essentials of teaching and learning in nursing ethics: Perspectives and methods*. London: Elsevier.

Drane, J. F. (1994). Character and the moral life. In E. R. DuBose, R. Hamel, & L. J. O'Connell (Eds.), *A matter of principles? ferment in U.S. bioethics* (pp. 284–309). Valley Forge, PA: Trinity Press International.

Frankena, W. K. (1973). *Ethics* (2nd ed.). Englewood Cliffs, NJ: Prentice-Hall.

Fry, S. T. (1989). Toward a theory of nursing ethics. *Advances in Nursing Science, 11*(4), 9–22.

Gert, B., Culver, C., & Clauser, K. (2006, March). Paternalism and its justification. *Bioethics, 47* 237–283.

Gilligan, C. (1993). *In a different voice: Psychological theory and women's development*. Cambridge, MA: Harvard University press.

Gudorf, C. E. (1994). A feminist critique of biomedical principlism. In E. R. Dubose, R. Hamel, & L. J. O'Connell (Eds.), *A matter of principles? Ferment in U.S. bioethics* (pp. 164–181). Valley Forge, PA: Trinity Press International.

Jonsen, A., & Butler, L. (1975). Public ethics and policy making. *The Hastings Center Report, 5*(4), 19–31.

Kant, I. (1964). *Groundwork of the metaphysics of morals.* J. Patton (Trans.) New York: Harper Perrenial.

Kant, I. (1965). *The metaphysical elements of justice: Part I of the metaphysics of morals.* Indianapolis: Bobbs-Merrill.

MacIntyre, A. (1966). *A short history of ethics.* New York: Macmillan.

MacIntyre, A. (1989). *Whose justice? Which rationality?* Notre Dame: University of Notre Dame.

Mill, J. S. (2002). In G. Sher (ed.), *Utilitarianism* (2nd ed.). New York: Hackett.

Morse, J. M., Bottorff, J., Neander, W., & Solberg, S. (1991). Comparative analysis of conceptualizations and theories of caring. *Image: The Journal of Nursing Scholarship, 23*(2), 119–126.

Nightingale, F. (2007). *Notes on nursing: What it is, and what it is not.* New York: Wilder Publications.

Noddings, N. (2003). *Caring: A feminine approach to ethics and moral education* (2nd ed.). Berkeley: University of California Press.

Rawls, J. (1971). *A theory of justice.* Cambridge, MA: Harvard University Press.

Rawls, J. (1999). *A theory of justice* (Chapter III). Cambridge, MA: Harvard University Press.

Rosen, F. (2003). *Classical utilitarianism from Hume to Mill.* London: Routledge.

Ross, W. D. (1970). What makes right acts right? In W. Sellars, & J. Hospers (Eds.), *Readings in ethical theory* (pp. 484–485). Englewood Cliffs, NJ: Prentice-Hall.

Ross, W. D. (2002). *The right and the good.* New York: Oxford University Press.

Sherwin, S. (1992). *No longer patient: Feminist ethics and health care.* Philadelphia, PA: Temple University Press.

CHAPTER 3

Nursing's Ethical Tradition: The 1870s to the Rise of Bioethics

Marsha Fowler

"Science fiction come alive" is an apt description of the development of medical science and technology since the late 1960s. Its astonishing miracles have also brought moral migraines for all who are or would be nurses or would seek the services of a nurse. As a consequence of the moral uncertainty, dilemmas, and distresses that contemporary health care has generated, and also as a response to the sometimes unwarranted and unwanted technologization of the end of life, the bioethical literature began to explode in that same period. Indeed, the expansion of bioethical literature, the creation of ethics centers, and the numbers of conferences, workshops, and intensive courses offered since the 1970s attest to the rise in importance of bioethical discourse in contemporary health care teaching, practice, and research.

Ethics has been the very foundation of nursing practice since the inception of modern nursing in the United States in the late 1870s. There is an unbroken thread of ethical literature and activity woven throughout the fabric of the entire profession—its literature, professional association, standards of practice (codes of ethics), educational requirements, position statements, and practice. Nothing within the profession has remained untouched by the enduring and intentional commitment to ethics. That commitment has included a massive ethical literature, attention to the ethical formation of the nursing student, development of a code of ethics, ongoing work of the American Nurses Association (ANA) in addressing ethical issues, and the formulation of ethical position statements with regard to health care and the role of the profession. The history of nursing's ethics is enduring, distinguished, honorable, and worthy of both our respect and pride.

THE NURSING ETHICAL LITERATURE

As nursing education began to move into the academy in the mid-1960s, the subsequent dissolution of the diploma schools' libraries has proven a substantial loss in the accessibility of early nursing ethical textbooks. Nonetheless, the extant literature is breathtaking in its intensity, commitment, insight, and compass.

Many of the textbooks, beginning with Isabel Robb's work, *Nursing Ethics: For Hospital and Private Use* (Robb, 1900b), went through several editions or were multiply reprinted. The works of Robb, Aikens (1916), Parsons (1916), and Talley (1925) (all nurse authors) were apparently particularly influential. Though somewhat misleading, nursing's ethics literature was sometimes published under the label "professional problems," "professional adjustments" (Dietz, 1935, 1940; Harrison, 1942) "the art of conduct," or even more obscurely as "friendly talks to nurses." Most of these books touched upon major aspects of the nurse's private and professional life.

Journal literature is equally impressive in volume and scope. *The Trained Nurse,* the first true journal of nursing, began in 1888. Commencing in May of 1889, the journal published a six-part series of articles on ethics in nursing. The articles divide "the duties of nursing into seven classes," each class being formed by a different relationship, for example, the nurse to the patient or the nurse to her friends.[1, 2] This relational motif for the discussion of the ethical duties of the nurse persists to this day. *The American Journal of Nursing (AJN),* which began in 1900, has also devoted considerable space to articles principally on ethics. In the October 1900 issue, an article by Isabel Robb describes a course of study that she recommends for those graduate nurses who would become superintendents of hospitals or schools of nursing. As one of the required subject areas for potential superintendents, Robb's article includes a section on nursing ethics, wherein she "levels" the content in terms of what should be taught to probationers, juniors, seniors, head nurses, and private duty nurses (Robb, 1900a). "Ethics in Nursing," by Isabel McIsaac, is the first *AJN* article actually devoted to ethics (McIsaac, 1900). Thereafter, from the first issue in 1900 to the early 1980s, the *AJN* has published over 400 articles principally devoted to ethics or topics in ethics (Fowler, 1984). Recognizing nurses' need for assistance with specific clinical-ethical problems, the *AJN* included a column entitled "Ethical problems," which ran from 1926 through 1928, stopped for 2 years, and then ran again from 1931 to 1934 (Committee on Ethical Standards, 1926). These columns solicit inquiries on ethical issues or problems in clinical practice from readers, to which the American Nurses Association Committee on Ethical Standards prepared and published a response. In addition, each of the Codes for Nurses has been published in the *AJN,* beginning with *A Suggested Code* in 1926 (American Nurses Association, 1926a).

The year 1935 marks the beginning of ethics research in nursing. In that year, Sr. Rose Helene Vaughn completed a "dissertation" (thesis) for the Master of Arts degree on *The Actual Incidence of Moral Problems in Nursing: A Preliminary Study In Empirical Ethics* at Catholic University of America (Vaughn, 1935). The results of the study indicated that the clinical-moral problem most frequently encountered by nurses was that of cooperation between nurses and physicians. It is not surprising that many of the moral problems encountered by nurses in 1935 persist. A case in point is her category "lust," which includes a number of incidents that today would be called "sexual harassment."

Given the extent of the early nursing ethical literature, ethics in nursing is no fad, but rather an enduring and intimate concern of the profession. To say this, however, is to give no indication of the nature and focus of ethics in nursing and its development to the present day. To understand nursing's ethics, it is necessary to have a closer look at the nursing ethical literature, tracing its evolution over the past 100 years.

THE FIRST HUNDRED YEARS OF ETHICS IN NURSING

Though it has been characterized as more concerned with etiquette than with ethics, this is to misunderstand early nursing ethics. Early nursing ethics focused on the character of the moral agent, refusing to separate personal from professional behavior. Despite being couched in the language of "good conduct," it was what the nurse *was*, not what the nurse *did*, that was important, the presumption being that good character would produce right action, that is, that virtue accomplished duty. Concerns for etiquette, then, were simply a part of the larger concern for right conduct as it emerged from right character. Thus, early nursing ethics texts contained sections on personal hygiene, physical self-care and recreation of the nurse, and even dating behaviors. The major emphases were, nonetheless, on more substantive concerns such as confidentiality. Nursing was a dominantly, sometimes exclusively, female profession. What was understood as "good conduct," "proper etiquette," and "right character" for nurses in the late 1800s and even into recent decades was always conditioned by what society understood to be the "proper" comportment and role of women in its day.

So, within the social context of 1900 and the social location of women in that day, what kind of a woman was the nurse to be? Robb quotes a letter she received asking for the recommendation of a nurse to fill a head-nurse position in a hospital that concludes, "in short, we require an intelligent saint" (Robb, 1900b). This does, in fact, capsulize Robb's understanding of the ideal nurse. It also contravenes the cultural norm of women as bearers of the "finer sensibilities" and men (not women) as the possessors of "intelligence." Indeed, higher education of women was culturally viewed as subversive of the species, as it was claimed to reduce female fertility, even to inducing withering of the reproductive organs. Nonetheless, Robb argues vigorously for the higher education of women as nurses (Robb, 1900b). Though her perspective would not particularly be seen as "feminist" today, in its time it was almost radically so.

Nursing students, particularly probationers and middle-year students, were generally seen to be morally unformed. The task of the nursing school was, therefore, in part, to shepherd the moral formation of the student, equipping the student for patient care, and for assuming a proper role in addressing the ills of society. The training school was about the business of shaping students into moral beings so that they could be trusted to deliver care as graduates, in unsupervised contexts. In addition, because the school was a place of moral formation, and because the emphasis was upon moral character, virtually the whole of the student's life was subject to moral scrutiny. Nursing was seen to be intelligent work, which was a view that ran countercurrent to societal perspectives on women. Students were to be morally equipped not simply with an ethics at the bedside, but also for a social ethics that addressed broader social problems. A quick look at nursing history will give ample evidence of nurses' involvement in causes related to child labor laws, public health, battles against poverty, leagues for animal protection, and a wide range of human and civil rights activism. Nursing's ethics is principally a social ethics that encompasses bioethics (Fowler, 1984).

Robb also holds that as nurses (including students) also exercise a moral influence upon patients, there is an additional burden in their moral formation. She writes that "only the character that is built on a foundation of generosity and sweetness (if linked to intelligence, common sense, and humor) is safe in any exigency that may arise. This character foundation is seldom inherited, but must be built up by training and practice" (Robb, 1900b). It was the task of the nursing school to undertake this training and practice.

How was the nurse to be toward the patient? Many of these ethics textbooks organize their discussion around the virtues, as learned attributes of moral character, seen as essential to the profession. But, overall, "to the patient laid low by disease or injury she appears as a goddess of healing, and her every gentle movement has a comforting and consoling power" (Goodrich, 1932). This "goddess of healing" nonetheless needed to be protected from certain evils; as a student, she was, it must be remembered, young, vulnerable, and not completely formed morally. Goodall writes "nursing will disclose the human body in conditions and circumstances that are new to your young eyes. There may be occasions when your only shield from the gross embarrassment will be your purity of mind" (Goodall, 1942). In 1947, priest-author McAllister writes more directly that:

> Duty sometimes *obliges* a person to think about things ordinarily dangerous to chastity. Medical students and nurses, to have the professional knowledge they need, must give considerable thought to matters of sex and processes of reproduction . . . they should guard against *morbid curiosity* and be cautious lest their studies become causes of *venereal pleasure.* (McAllister, 1947/1955)

The education necessary to care for patients who might have questions or problems with sex or reproduction posed a grievous moral danger to the nurse. Note that this perspective (found also in the later 1955 edition of McAllister's work) occurs relatively late within the context of the social shifts in society regarding sexual matters. Yet, sex and reproductive education are not the only danger confronting the student and from which the student might need protection. In 1943, Goodall writes:

> In dormitory life or in any other way of life, avoid crushes for they will rob you of all healthy, natural desire to mingle with groups of people and within your life they will harbor evils and miseries that jealousy can bring. When carried too far, they will turn your emotions from their natural bent and cause you to have an unnatural and unhappy attitude toward men . . . the best rule in friendship is to be fond of many and familiar with none. (Goodall, 1942)

This expression of homophobia reflected a prevailing though covert fear that women living together in close quarters, as nursing students were required to do, would form emotional attachments that might "turn [their] emotions from their natural bent and cause" them to become lesbian. Students needed to be protected until they could develop the strength of moral character to weather the moral assaults of sex education, living in close quarters with other women, dating, the advances made by male patients or patient relatives, or physicians, and the temptations of extravagance with one's wages. The world of the nursing student was seen to be rife with potentially corrupting influences from which the student had paternalistically to be protected.

The emphasis on the character of the moral agent, otherwise known as "virtue ethics," was not unique to nursing, but rather reflected the prevailing societal perspective on ethics. However, the emphasis on the moral purity of the nurse endures beyond the point at which society ceases to embrace an ethics that allows scrutiny of the personal life, particularly of public figures. That is to say, long after society began to shift toward a duty-based ethics, nursing retained an emphasis on virtue ethics. This may in part be due to the nature of nursing education, which took place in essentially cloistered contexts similar to Erving Goffman's "total institution" (Goffmann, 1961). The virtues considered essential to the character of the nurse, those that made for a "morally good nurse," the virtues and excellences reflected in the ethical literature of the past 100 years, included among many others such "virtues" as cleanliness, cheerfulness, gentler virtues, good breeding, good posture, good grammar, high thinking, humanitarianism, industri-ousness, long suffering, loyal, neatness, meekness, joyfulness, tenderheartedness, resistance to infection, uncomplaining, unobtrusiveness, wholesomeness, and perfect womanliness (Fowler, 1984).

True virtues or excellences expected of the nurse in days past (as opposed to cultural expectations of women) include benevolence, care, compassion, competence, courage, devotion, faithfulness, honesty, integrity, justness, kindness, knowledgeable, loving, loyal, nonmalevolent, prudent, skilled, teachable, temperate, tolerant, trustwor-thy, wise, understanding, and truthful (Fowler, 1984). This is, in fact, a sound reflection of the moral attributes that one would hope to see in nurses today.

In the late 1960s, nursing, following societal changes and heavily influenced by the rise of the field of bioethics, shifted away from a virtue-based ethics to a duty-based ethics. Yet, it is not an "either–or" situation, but rather a "both–and" necessity. Both a virtue and a duty-based approach to ethics is essential if duties are to have any power and if virtues are to have any direction. The problem of a duty-based ethics is that obligations are empty if the person does not possess the moral character to meet those obligations. The problem of a virtue-based ethics is that it runs the risk of abuse through unwarranted intrusion into the private life of the individual, an intrusion that was amply evident in our early isolated "live-in education." Nursing needs to avoid any return to such abuses. However, it also needs to reclaim the importance of virtue ethics, not for the purposes of the moral examination of the practitioner, but rather for the scrutiny of the environment in which care is rendered (De Raeve, 2006). That environment needs to nurture virtues and to allow them to flourish. For example, can the virtues of knowledge, skill, patience, and caring flourish in an environment where the nurse's patient load is so large that competence and safety are the surpassing concerns? Where the practice environment mitigates against the exercise of specific virtues or excellences, it is inappropriate to demand or expect them.

CODES OF ETHICS FOR NURSING

The Nightingale Pledge

Though never formally adopted as a code of ethics for the profession, THE Florence Nightingale Pledge was influential for generations of nurses. It was penned by Lystra Gretter of the Farrand School of Nursing in Detroit in 1893. The story of the Pledge and its subsequent revision in 1935 is interesting. The original Pledge is:

> I solemnly pledge myself before God and in the presence of this assembly, to pass my life in purity and to practice my profession faithfully. I will abstain from whatever is deleterious and mischievous, and will not take or knowingly administer any harmful drug. I will do all in my power to

maintain and elevate the standard of my profession, and will hold in confidence all personal matters committed to my keeping, and all family affairs coming to my knowledge in the practice of my calling. With loyalty will I endeavor to aid the physician in his work, and devote myself to the welfare of those committed to my care.[3]

The revised Pledge reads as follows:

I solemnly pledge myself before God and in the presence of this assembly to pass my life in purity and to practice my profession faithfully. I will abstain from whatever is deleterious and mischievous, and will not take or knowingly administer any harmful drug. I will do all in my power to maintain and elevate the standard of my profession, and will hold in confidence all personal matters committed to my keeping, and all family affairs coming to my knowledge in the practice of my calling. With loyalty will I endeavor to aid the physician in his work, and as a "missioner of health" I will dedicate myself to devoted service to human welfare.[4]

An accompanying note, written on Farrand School letterhead in Gretter's own hand reads as follows:

Commensurate with the broader activities of the Farrand Training School of Nurses The Florence Nightingale Pledge has been revised to include service to the community within its scope. [signed] Lystra E. Gretter[5]

The story of its origin and revision is as detailed in the following note (quoted in its entirety) from the archives of the Alumnae Association of the Farrand Training School for Nurses.[6]

ORIGIN OF THE FLORENCE NIGHTINGALE PLEDGE

In 1893, two years after Mrs. L. E. Gretter came to the Farrand Training School for Nurses (now the Harper Hospital School of Nursing) as Principal and because Florence Nightingale was her ideal of what a professional nurse should be, that she conceived the idea that young women engaged in nursing needed something similar to the Hippocratic Oath, and she presented her idea to the Board of Trustees of Harper Hospital, which appointed a committee of three, namely:

Mrs. Gretter–chairman
N.E.H. Haight–Supervisor
Louise Tempest Ford–Supervisor
Dr. W.H. Davis–D.D.

Mrs. Gretter was appointed to draft a tentative pledge, as she had in mind, and when presented to the Board of Trustees for consideration, it was accepted without change.

At the time, Mrs. Gretter had only the graduates of the School in mind and it is administered to the graduates at their graduating exercises every year.

During the World War I, through the influence of Mrs. Gretter, and as a war measure, it was decided to by the various schools of nursing in Detroit, to combine the commencement exercises, and at that time Mrs. Gretter was invited to administer the Florence Nightingale Pledge to the group.

This had the effect of making the Pledge generally known, and it was not long before advertising firms, book publishers, and many others using it for profit, until in 1933, while the material was being assembled for the "School"—when several of the graduates considered that it was time to do something to protect the Pledge. Agnes G. Deans made a special trip to the Department of Copyright in Washington, and took up the question of having it copyrighted. When the facts were considered, it was found that the time had expired between the time the Pledge had been formulated, and at that time (1933) but the clerk suggested that if Mrs. Gretter was willing to make a slight revision that it could be copyrighted.[7] Mrs. Gretter did, and this was incorporated in the "History of the Farrand Training School," which was incorporated.

As the sale of the History of the School was rather limited, this information did not get over to the public, and the commercial purposes for which it had been used, continued. Another trip was made to Washington by Miss Deans to determine what could be done, and was assured that the pledge was protected by law. As part of the history, and it was suggested that some wider publicity be given the fact.

An appeal was made to the *American Journal of Nursing*, and the *Pacific Coast Journal of Nursing*, and the *Trained Nurse and Hospital Review* for some publicity, which was given. This helped very much. (See correspondence on file under "Nightingale Pledge.")[8]

The Nightingale Pledge (1893) was well received across the country and continued to be administered at graduation exercises nationwide long after the ANA adopted a formal Code for Nurses in 1950.

THE DEVELOPMENT OF AN OFFICIAL CODE OF ETHICS FOR THE PROFESSION

Three years after the creation of the Pledge, delegates and representatives of the American Society of Superintendents of Training Schools for Nurses convened to establish a professional association for nurses and to write its articles of incorporation. The Nurses' Associated Alumnae of the United States and Canada (later the ANA and the Canadian Nurses' Associations) was formed at that meeting. In the articles of incorporation, they identify their purposes, the first of which is "to establish and maintain a code of ethics."[9] It was then another 53 years before a code of ethics was officially adopted. Before it could address the need for a code, nursing would need to deal with issues of mandatory uniform registration, the evaluation and accreditation of nursing schools, and a number of issues affecting the economic and general welfare of nurses. So, preparation of a code was delayed.

There was, however, continuing demand for a code of ethics, to the degree that, in 1921, the National League of Nursing Education (NLNE) appointed an advisory

Committee on Ethical Standards. The Committee studied the need for a code of ethics for the profession and concluded that "nurses throughout the country are desiring something concrete which they may accept as a basis for professional conduct" (Powell, 1923). The committee formally recommended the preparation of a "statement of the principles of nursing ethics" (ANA, 1924). The NLNE received and approved the recommendations of the report. However, at a meeting of the joint boards of the NLNE and the ANA held in 1923, the ANA president (Adda Eldrege) requested that the committee become a part of the ANA rather than the NLNE. The reason given was that the ANA "had planned to compile a code of ethics as a part of the Association's work" (ANA, 1926b). Thus, the actual task of preparing a code of ethics was shifted to the ANA.

The ANA committee met in 1923 and after study and discussion concluded that "inasmuch as nursing ideals had been for so many years so beautifully expressed by members of the profession, it seems to us undesirable at this time to outline the elementary principles of good conduct as the code of ethics endorsed by the American Nurses Association" (ANA, 1924). The committee recommended, instead, "a restatement of these high ideals in form somewhat similar to that of the Fellowship Pledge of the American College of Surgeons" (ANA, 1924). However, in January of 1926, a subcommittee presented a proposed code to the parent committee. Suggestions for emendation were then made by the joint boards of directors of the ANA and NLNE, with the recommendation that the amended version be published in the *AJN* as an "editorial," soliciting opinions and suggestions from the readership. The joint boards accepted and approved the code with the provision that it be identified as a preliminary or tentative code (ANA, 1924).

A Suggested Code was published in the August 1926 issue of the *AJN* (ANA, 1926a). (It was also at this point that the Committee decided to institute the *AJN* column "Ethical Problems.") Written in the rhetorically effusive style of the late 1800s and early 1900s, the 1926 code was never formally adopted. It discussed the moral duties of the nurse, organizing its discussion around the various relationships nurses form; specific principles of ethics were not enumerated. Part of the importance of this code, however, resides in its specification of the central moral motif of nursing: *the ideal of service*. The language is stylistically excessive but essentially accurate: "the most precious possession of this profession is the ideal of service, extending even to the sacrifice of life itself" (ANA, 1926a). This ideal of service links all the disparate historical forms of nursing into a contiguous whole and finds its distinctive "local" expression in metaphors of each day. For instance, the ideal of service today is expressed in the metaphor of caring, a metaphor that would not have been an adequate expression in earlier eras, for example, the nursing Knights Templar.

In 1940, *A Tentative Code* was published (ANA, 1940). It retains the relational format of the 1926 Code and demonstrates a more overt concern for the status of nursing as a profession and for the public recognition of nursing. This Code lists the attributes of a profession and argues for the status of nursing as a profession; unfortunately, this is subject matter that does not properly belong in a code of ethics. Responses were sought from the *AJN* readers following the publication of the 1926 and 1940 codes. The responses were partly responsible for the reformulation of the 1940 Code in 1949. The reformulated Code was presented to ANA members, schools of nursing, and health care institutions. Input was also solicited through a questionnaire mailed to individuals (that resulted in replics representing 4,759 persons). The *Code for Professional Nurses* was accepted, unanimously, at the 1950 ANA House of Delegates. At last, the profession had an official code of ethics (Fowler, 1992).

The 1950 Code differs dramatically in style from its predecessors. It has a brief preamble and enumerates 17 provisions. The provisions are organized around the relational pattern of previous codes, though this pattern is not made explicit. Several provisions relate to the personal ethics (private life) of the nurse. A formal code of ethics is not a static document; it requires periodic revision (probably every 8 to 10 years) in order to keep abreast of changes in clinical practice and in society. While the principles may not themselves change, new situations arise in which they must be applied.

In 1957, a minor change was made to the Code in relation to nurse participation in advertising. Nursing was deeply concerned in this period to establish itself as a legitimate "profession" with all the rights and privileges appertaining thereto. As a consequence, it adopted some norms of other groups that society regarded as professions. A case in point is the adoption of a provision against advertising, a long-held norm maintained by both medicine and law. Historically, however, the reason not to advertise services was to prevent fee wars that would drive down the income of the professional. This was usually sanitized for public consumption by declaring that the prohibition against advertising protected the public from quackery. In the 1950s, television used "nurses" (dramatized) in advertising, initiating a flurry of protest and communications. When inquiry was made about the nursing Code's proscription of advertising, the response was that it was for the protection of the public. However, the specific products in question were Mum deodorant and Bromo-Seltzer. It is not always the case that all the provisions of professional codes are well grounded in ethical reasoning; codes must always be evaluated for their degree of legitimate self-interest over against self-protectionism (Fowler, 1984). It must be added that nursing's history, and its codes, are remarkably free of self-interest, sometimes perhaps too much so.

Following the adoption of the Code in 1950, responses were again solicited from *AJN* readers. These responses formed the basis of the 1960 major revision of the *Code*. The *Code* of 1960 reflects the social context of increasing assertiveness of nursing and nurses and an increasing sense of coparticipation (rather than subordination) of nurses in the care of patients. From the vantage point of the 1990s, this Code has a greater sense of professional freedom. Between 1950 and 1960, concern arose regarding the enforcement of the *Code*. The ANA bylaws were subsequently revised to include the obligations of members to uphold the Code. By 1964, the Committee on Ethics developed *Suggested Guidelines for Handling Violations of the Code for Professional Nurses* and distributed them to each affiliate state and territorial association.

The next major revision of the *Code* was published in 1968. This revision omits the preamble of the 1960 Code and reduces the number of provisions from 17 to 10. For the most part, however, it encompasses all of the concerns of the *Code* of 1960. As this Code provides the basis of the provisions of the 1976 and 1985 revised codes, there has effectively been no revision of the provisions of the Code themselves for 33 years (until the Code of 2001), though revisions in the interpretive statements have been made.

One of the more significant changes in the Code of 1968 is its omission, for the first time, of any reference to the private behavior of the nurse. A wedge is driven between private and professional ethics, when the 1968 *Code* drops the expectation that the nurse "would adhere to standards of personal ethics which reflect credit upon the profession" (Fowler, 1992). Nursing now fully moves into a duty-based ethics, leaving behind much of its traditional ethical focus on virtue.

In the 1970s, changes in nursing, medicine, and society made another revision of the *Code* necessary. The revised *Code* was published in 1976, giving greater emphasis to the responsibilities of the patient to participate in her or his care. The *Code for Nurses,* 1976, was published with *Interpretive Statements* that interpret the provisions in the light of contemporary nursing and health care and professional concerns. It is in this code that the term *patient* is changed to *client.* This Code makes some modest revision to the 1968 *Code* itself, in accord with an increased social consciousness regarding forms of prejudicial discrimination, an increased technologization of the clinical arena, an increased awareness of medical paternalism, and an increased autonomy (and freedom) of nurses. It also gives increased emphasis to the nurse's responsibility and accountability in the relationship with the patient and, overall, takes a more assertive and activistic posture with regard to the nurse and the nursing profession. The streamlining of the language of this Code leads to a parsimony that stands in great contrast to the effusiveness and rhetorical elegance of the earliest codes. Nonetheless, it is a more fulsome and professionally energetic code.

In 1985, again in response to changes within the profession, in medicine and medical technology, and in society, another revision was published. This *Code* retains, intact, the provisions of the 1976 *Code* and many of that code's categories, but changes the *Interpretive Statements* to reflect the concerns of the day. The 1985 *Code,* more than any previous *Code,* attends to the changes that were occurring in the field of bioethics both in relation to specific issues and in relation to professional behavior in general. It relies heavily, too much so, upon a principled approach to ethical analysis and decision making. It also, appropriately, takes a more ethical approach, purging some of the legal language of previous codes. This *Code* has a heightened awareness of more subtle forms of unjust societal discrimination, of the unwarranted and unwanted intrusion of medical care and the technologization of the end of life, of poor access to care, of the nurse's ever-expanding role as advocate for health, both for individuals and for society. In 1995, the ANA, through its center for Ethics and Human Rights, convened a task force to examine the *Code* and to make a recommendation as to whether the *Code* or its interpretive statements needed revision, in whole or in part. The task force recommended that the ANA undertake a revision of both the *Code* itself, that is, the provisions themselves, which has not been revised since 1976, and its *Interpretive Statements.* A Code of Ethics Project Task Force of ten persons was appointed to begin work on the *Code* and its interpretive statements in late 1996.

In 2001, the work of the Task Force came to fruition when the new *Code of Ethics for Nurses* was adopted by the House of Delegates at the ANA biennial meeting (ANA, 2001). This *Code* is a substantially revised document: Both the provisions of the Code and the interpretive statements underwent major revision. To summarize, this *Code* is more broadly based in the field of ethics, rather than relying almost exclusively upon a principled approach to ethics. Work in virtue, caring, feminist, and communitarian ethics, in particular, has been taken into account. The contemporary clinical environment is economically tense and tends to assert a priority of business values over those of nursing in general or caring in particular; this had profound ramifications for the way in which health care proceeds ethically. This tension is reflected in the interpretive statements of the 2001 *Code*. Moreover, the potential for moral harm to the nurse in this kind of environment (by preventing the fulfillment of moral duties or the growth of virtues and excellences) was of substantial importance to the Task Force, which was concerned to demand in all nursing contexts a moral milieu consistent with human flourishing and excellence of nursing practice. The new *Code* reflects an increasing sense of world community, not just national identity; that is, it is more globalizing. It is also more aggressive regarding nursing responsibility to challenge and work to correct the social ills that mitigate against access to care, that foster disease, illness, or trauma, and that see personal health as separate from urban or social health. The new interpretive statements also narrow the wedge that has been driven between personal and professional ethics; one cannot be a rogue and scoundrel in private life and yet a public person of integrity and moral rectitude (ANA, 2001).

Specific changes to the Code include the following (ANA, 2001):

- Changing the title to *Code of Ethics*
- Broadening of the Code to include all nurses in all positions, not limiting the *Code* to nurses in clinical practice
- A recombination of the 11 provisions of the Code of 1985 into 7 provisions and the addition of two wholly new provisions (5 and 9)
- Greater attention to "rights," the problems of "delegation" of nursing tasks, the "health care environment," and "conditions of employment"
- The bold assertion that the nurse's primary commitment is to the *patient*
- The inclusion of duties to self, that is, the duties that a nurse has to herself or himself
- The recognition that the advance of the profession comes through several avenues, and not solely through research
- A greater emphasis on the international, global nature of health
- A statement on the collective moral responsibility of nurses, as exercised through professional associations
- A section afterward incorporated into the document that discusses briefly the development of the Code and its evolution.

The new Code of Ethics for Nurses with Interpretive Statements is a remarkable document that is best appreciated through careful reading of both this and the preceding *Code*. This reading in tandem will highlight not only the changes in the *Code* per se, but will also spotlight the changes in the context of nursing and health care for American nurses.

A code of ethics, if it is to serve the profession in maintaining the standards of the profession, must reflect both constancy and change. It must reflect constancy in its commitment to the central values of the profession, its central moral motif of service, its emphasis upon social as well as "bedside" ethics, and its enduring moral tradition. It must reflect change in its application to ever-new clinical and professional concerns, moral insights and awarenesses, changes in professional knowledge and role, and social change. Though the norms themselves are stable, they must be reinterpreted afresh for each generation of nurses in accordance with the growth of the profession and changes in society.

Nursing's ethics has a long, distinctive, and distinguished history, demonstrating an enduring and intimate concern for the ethical practice of nurses and for the well-being of society. That concern for ethics has suffused its literature, its education, its practice, and its research. The Code for Nurses, rooted in the tradition of the Nightingale Pledge, is almost 100 years old. Along the way, nursing has spoken out in society through moral position statements, through testimony before Congress, through its Code, and through its work to seek to achieve health for all. The nursing ethical tradition is one of which we can be enormously proud.

Notes

1. HCC (Otherwise unidentified superintendent of a Brooklyn school of nursing): "The Ethics of Nursing." *The Trained Nurse,* Vol. II, 5:179. The remaining articles of the series are found in Volume III, No. 1–6.
2. By convention extant literature, irrespective of the date it was first written, is properly referred to in the present tense.
3. Gretter, L. E. *The florence nightingale pledge.* Detroit: Farrand Training School for Nurses, Harper Hospital. Taken from a photograph of the original autograph manuscript (original was discovered to have been removed from the archival scrapbook), dated April 30, 1893. Photograph of original manuscript dates from before 1929. *Used with permission.*
4. Gretter, L. E. *The Florence Nightingale Pledge.* Taken from autograph manuscript, dated January 1, 1936. *Used with permission.*
5. Gretter, L. E. Autograph note on letterhead of Harper Hospital, Farrand Training School for Nurses, Principal's Office. Dated January 1, 1936. *Used with permission.*
6. Anonymous. From the files of Harper Hospital School of Nursing. Paper typed and hand dated "c. 1938," quoted en toto with spelling and punctuation left uncorrected. *Used with permission.*
7. Ibid.
8. Ibid.
9. Convention of Training School Alumnae Delegates and Representatives from the American Society of Superintendents of Training Schools for Nurses (1896). *Proceedings of the Convention, 2–4 November 1896.* Harrisburg: Harrisburg Publishing.

References

Aikens, C. A. (1916). *Studies in ethics for nurses.* Philadelphia: W.B. Saunders.

American Nurses Association (ANA). (1924). Report of the committee on ethical standards. *Minutes of the Proceedings of the 24th Convention of the American Nurses Association.* New York: American Nurses Association.

American Nurses Association (ANA). (1926a). A suggested code. *The American Journal of Nursing, 26*(8), 599–601.

American Nurses Association (ANA). (1926b). Report of the committee on ethical standards. *Minutes of the Proceedings of the 25th Convention of the American Nurses Association.* New York: American Nurses Association.

American Nurses Association (ANA). (2001). *The code of ethics for nurses with interpretive statements.* Silver Spring, MD: ANA.

American Nurses Association (ANA). (1940). A tentative code. *The American Journal of Nursing, 40*(9), 977–980.

Committee on Ethical Standards. (1926). American nurses association: Ethical problems. *The American Journal of Nursing, 26*(8), 643.

De Raeve, L. (2006). Virtue ethics. In A. Davis, V. Tschudin, & L. de Rarve (Eds.), *Essentials of teaching and learning ethics: Perspectives and methods* (pp. 97–108). London: Chruchill Livingstone/Elsevier.

Dietz, L. D. (1935). *Professional problems in nursing*. Philadelphia: F.A. Davis.

Dietz, L. D. (1940). *Professional Adjustments, I*. Philadelphia: F.A. Davis.

Fowler, M. (1984). *Ethics in nursing, 1893–1984: The ideal of service, the reality of history*. Los Angeles: University of Southern California.

Fowler, M. (1992). A chronicle of the evolution of the code for nurses. In G. White (Ed.), *Ethical dilemmas in contemporary nursing practice* (pp. 149–154). Washington, DC: American Nurses Association.

Goffmann, E. (1961). *Asylums*. New York: Anchor.

Goodall, P. A. (1942). *Ethics: The inner realities*. Philadelphia, PA: F.A. Davis. (Also 1943.)

Goodrich, A. W. (1932). *The social and ethical significance of nursing: A series of addresses*. New York: Macmillan.

Harrison, H. (1942). *Professional adjustments*. No publisher given.

McAllister, J. B. (1947). *Ethics with special application to the medical and nursing professions*. Philadelphia, PA: W.B. Saunders. (Also 1955.)

McIsaac, I. (1900). Ethics in nursing. *The American Journal of Nursing, 1*(7), 488–490.

Parsons, S. E. (1916). *Nursing problems and obligations*. Boston: Whitcomb and Barrows. (Also, 1919, 1922.)

Powell, L. (1923). Report of the committee on ethical standards. *NLNE: Proceedings of the 28th Annual convention, Seattle Washington, June 26–July 1, 1922* (pp. 27–28). Baltimore: Williams & Wilkins.

Robb, I. A. H. (1900a). Hospital economics. *The American Journal of Nursing, 1*(1), 29–36.

Robb, I. A. H. (1900b). *Nursing ethics: For hospital and private use*. New York: E.C. Koeckert. (Reprinted without revision in 1911, 1916, 1920.)

Talley, C. E. (1925). *Ethics: A textbook for nurses*. New York: Putnam's. (2nd ed. 1928.)

Vaughn, S. R. H. (1935). *The actual incidence of moral problems in nursing: A preliminary study in empirical ethics*. Washington, DC: Catholic University Press.

CHAPTER 4

Professional Ethics and Institutional Constraints in Nursing Practice

THE IMPORTANCE OF NURSING: SOME FACTS

The Bureau of Labor Statistics reports that there are nearly 2.9 million registered nurses (RNs) in the United States and 2.4 million of them are actively employed. This report also indicates that nursing is number one on the list of the top 10 growth occupations. However, the trend of nurses retiring or leaving the profession and not enough new nurses being prepared has led to a shortage. The prediction is that the number of RNs will fall 20 percent below the demand by 2010.[1]

Schools of nursing are turning away applicants in large numbers due to the shortage of nurse educators. The Congressional Nursing Caucus, a bipartisan initiative, was formed in 2003 to educate members of Congress on all aspects of nursing and how nursing impacts the delivery of quality, safe care. For example, they are told that research indicates that advanced practice RNs can provide 60–80 percent of primary care as well as or better than physicians and at a lesser cost. These nurses can legally prescribe medications (American Nurses Association, 2008). According to numerous recent annual Gallup Polls, nurses rank first or second for their honesty and integrity, with 82 percent of Americans rating them high or very high.[2]

So why, if nursing is so important to the well-being of the country and nurses are consistently ranked high in virtues by the public, do nurses face constraints that sometimes make it difficult for them to be ethical? This chapter focuses on that question.

Specifically, this chapter discusses the nature of professional ethics in nursing and some of the institutional and social constraints that can act to inhibit the ethical practice of nursing, along with recent developments that attempt to lessen or eliminate these constraints. The discussion will be generally focused on U.S. nurses who practice in hospitals because we have more data on them. Nursing is the largest health care occupation, with 59 percent of nursing positions located in hospitals.[3]

MULTIPLE ETHICAL OBLIGATIONS/RESPONSIBILITIES

The overriding ethical issue for nurses, especially those working in hospitals, can best be described as one of multiple ethical obligations coupled with the question of authority. As professionals, nurses have a moral code that maintains that their primary ethical obligation is to the patient. This, in general, means that when an ethical dilemma arises, the nurse places the patient at the center of the dilemma and seeks to discover the patient's ethical position based on his or her deeply held values. The main question is this: What does the patient think is the right thing for him or her in this situation? In some ethical dilemmas, nurses simply want to replace the physician's ethical stance with their own, without either the physician or the nurses having full knowledge of the patient's ethical stance.

Nurses have an ethical obligation to the patient, but they also have an ethical obligation to the physician and to the institution in which they work. As professionals, nurses owe their primary ethical obligation to the patient; however, as employees, nurses also have ethical obligations to the employing institution and the physician. To the extent that these multiple ethical obligations mesh so that no conflict develops among them, the nurse should have a clear idea of the right action to take. However, when conflicts arise between or among these ethical obligations, the nurse faces an ethical dilemma.

Several examples will help in better understanding the concept of multiple obligations. If the physician makes the decision to withhold information about Mr. Brown's diagnosis and prognosis on the basis of his or her best clinical judgment, but the nurses, in their best clinical judgment, believe that Mr. Brown should be given this information so that he may function morally as an autonomous person, the ethical dilemma involving multiple obligations has occurred. Should the nurses go along with the physician and support the decision to withhold information or should they attempt to change the situation so that Mr. Brown will know his health status and be able to plan his life accordingly? It will make a difference if there is evidence that Mr. Brown does or does not want to know this information.

Further, what should the nurse, Ms Hyde, do in a situation where information has been withheld or distorted by the hospital authorities to prevent a legal suit by the patient's family when a mistake was made in surgery? If the family knows this information, they may sue, and such a legal suit, if won, can hurt the hospital's reputation and financial stability. Should Ms Hyde go along with the hospital's definition of events that transpired in the operating room because of her obligation to her employer or should she attempt to have the patient's family told what really happened? What is the ethical thing to do regarding this patient? What is the common good and should it be considered?

Ethical decisions are usually made in a social context, and that context often has within it potential constraints that make taking an ethical stance and acting on it a complex matter. The physician has a special legal relationship with the patient, whereas the nurse's legal obligations vary according to a state's nurse-practice act. This fact makes nursing ethics more complex in clinical settings. This social reality of ethics makes being ethical both more difficult in many situations and more complicated. Ethical obligations may go beyond what is legally required, but ethics does not often ask individuals to break the law. The simple answer to this problem is that the nurse should do what is right and abide by the ANA *Code of Ethics for Nurses*. However, an examination of any dilemma of multiple ethical obligations brings into sharp focus the fact that answers to ethical dilemmas are not always so easily derived.

In the first example given above, the nurse must make a choice between the physician's decision to withhold information and the patient's right to have this information. Let us assume that the physician's stance is based on the ethical principles of nonmaleficence (do no harm) and beneficence (do good) and that he or she believes that to tell Mr. Brown would do harm, since Mr. Brown does not seem emotionally able to cope with the facts of his case. Suppose that Mr. Brown has indicated to the nurse that he has some questions about his illness and wonders if he has been told the facts. The nurse, then, becomes concerned about the ethical principle of respect for autonomy as well as the meaning of caring in relationship with Mr. Brown and wonders if withholding information from this patient is ethically wrong. The nurse then believes that the patient should be told. Both the nurse and the physician are acting to meet what they think is their ethical obligation to the patient. Yet, it is the nurse who confronts a situation of multiple ethical obligations, obligations to both the patient and the physician. This is complicated by the fact that the physician is viewed as having more authority to make this type of decision because of the physician's role, social stature, and clinical judgment.

When nurses confront situations involving multiple ethical obligations, the first question is this: What is the right thing to do, and in what ways can I think about this problem that may help me to know what the right action is? Along with this question, another one comes into play: How far does the nurse's ethical obligation extend? If, in this situation the nurse reasons that the right thing to do is to withhold information, there is no problem of multiple ethical obligations. However, if the nurse does not agree with this decision to withhold information, the second question arises: How far and in what directions does the nurse pursue this obligation to the patient? Should the nurse tell Mr. Brown his diagnosis and prognosis? One can argue that this is the ethical and legal obligation of the physician. What if the nurse goes to the physician and explains that Mr. Brown is asking for information about his diagnosis and that she thinks the physician should talk with Mr. Brown about this? What if the physician continues with the decision to withhold the information even after the nurse has given these additional data? Has the nurse met the ethical obligation to Mr. Brown? Should the nurse go to other persons or committees, and, if so, which ones? Suppose the nurse goes to the head nurse, but the head nurse does nothing about the situation. Has the nurse's ethical obligation been met? All of these and similar concerns stem from several questions that nurses need to think about:

1. What is the nurse's ethical obligation in those situations of multiple ethical obligations?
2. What is the extent of these obligations?
3. What ethically ought the relationship between the nurse and the patient be?
4. What does it mean to be a virtuous person in this situation?
5. What is caring, as defined in nursing, in this situation?

NURSING ROLES AND ETHICS—HISTORICAL BACKGROUND

Many books on nursing ethics in the past have in large part restricted their content to professional etiquette. In 1900, the early nursing leader Isabel Robb wrote of a breach of etiquette and her comments reflect the sociology of the situation of that day, including differences in role, function, and status. She remarked that occasionally we find a nurse who, through ignorance or from an increase of her self-conceit and an exaggerated idea of her importance, may overstep the boundary in her relationship with the doctor and commit some breach of etiquette. Robb said that not only will the individual nurse be made to suffer most acutely, but also her school and the profession at large come in for a share of criticism and blame (Robb, 1900). Aikens, in 1937, devoted two chapters to what she called old-fashioned virtues and included truth in nursing reports, discreetness of speech, obedience, being teachable, respect for authority, discipline, and loyalty (Aikens, 1937).

One of the most interesting books in the 1940s on nursing ethics had a chapter entitled "Master and Servant: Physicians and Nurse." It says that if the hospital employs the nurse, she is a servant of the hospital and as such the hospital becomes responsible for her acts. With this status, any disobedience to the physician's orders is not only a matter of professional etiquette, but a violation of the employee contract. In those situations in which the nurse knows that the physician is mishandling the patient's treatment, she must either continue to carry out his orders or give up the case. The author points out that the nurse has no duty to enlighten the public on the relative merits of physicians and the value of their treatment. In short, the nurse ought to remember that she has "a duty of charity as a faithful servant to a master to protect the good name and reputation of the physician under whom she works" (Moore, 1943).

In the 1950s, another author quoted a remark made by a physician to a nursing school graduating class—he said that to be a successful nurse, one must also be a successful liar. This quote led the book's author into a discussion of loyalty as the nurse's first duty. By virtue of her profession as well as of her implied contract, the nurse owes the physician not only efficient care of patients but also such evidence of loyalty as will strengthen the patient's confidence in him (McAllister, 1955).

All of these references on nursing ethics were written in the 20th century. Such input reflects the nature of the socialization process into nursing, the role of women and nurses, the physician's role, and the hierarchical organization in hospitals. Many of these early ethics books delved into the private life and morality of nurses, reflecting the status of nursing students in an apprenticeship system and the stereotype of the intellectually and morally weak woman. Such concerns focused on the individual nurse's morality and the nurse's duties, obligations, and loyalties. Nurses were, on the one hand, expected to exhibit a dedication of almost a religious nature, while, on the other hand, their morality was open to suspicion. Remnants of this legacy remain today because some types of change come slowly due to multiple complex social and economic factors.

More recently, a multinational research project has asked questions about the value of nursing (Horton, 2007). That this question is being asked in 2008 implies that nursing has some enduring professional issues (D'Antonio, Baer, Rinker, & Lynaugh, 2006). Such issues as professional role, gender, education, public image, work environment, and status are central to nursing history and its present situation in which ethical dilemmas occur.

MORAL DISTRESS

In 2001, the ANA conducted a staffing survey in which nurses said that deteriorating working conditions have led to dissatisfaction regarding the level of care possible in present hospital work environments.[4] Given the gap between expectations of the nursing profession and of individual nurses and the realities of the workplace, nurses can experience moral distress. That is, often nurses know what should be done but due to these external factors they believe that they cannot act on their knowledge and professional values. One of the aims of this book is to provide nurses with ways of thinking about and addressing these organizational and social constraints that create moral distress.

Once of the earliest references to moral distress experienced by nurses was discussed by Jameton (1984). Over the last 25 years, numerous articles written by nurses on this topic can be found in many journals, including the international journal *Nursing Ethics*.[5]

A recent book of essays in which nurses speak out about physicians presents a mixed bag of experiences but indicates that the relationship between nurses and physicians is important to both as they work in the same constraining environment (Ratner, 2008). The business model that permeates much of American health care today creates clinical and ethical issues for both nurses and doctors. The United States is the only industrialized country in the world without a national health care system. While education is valued as a right for all in America, health care is not. Two major issues in the 2008 presidential election were the economy and health care. While this book mainly discusses nurses working in hospitals, it is important to remember that many citizens have no health care insurance and so never become hospital patients. This is a problem in the ethical principle of justice. Moral distress can be experienced by any nurse, including those working in hospitals, in community health, and in free clinics for those citizens who do not have health care insurance.

DYNAMICS AND LOYALTIES

As mentioned earlier, one of the most interesting dimensions of hospital nursing arises in the potential for conflicting moral claims or multiple ethical obligations of the nurse. All nurses from top administrators to staff find themselves in situations involving multiple ethical obligations. Until around the time of World War II, many, if not most, nurses in hospitals worked as private duty nurses there and in the home and received a fee for their services from the patient. A number of economic and sociological factors converged in the 1930s and 1940s, and a shift away from fee for service to hospital–employee status occurred. Whereas previously the nurse's obligation had been to the one patient and the patient's physician, with this shift came a change in occupational status, and the ethics of the situation became more complex. As a hospital employee, the nurse must now balance obligations to the institution, to the attending physician and the house staff, and to the patients themselves, while attempting to practice nursing using the ethics code of the profession as a guideline.

In the past, nurses believed that their first loyalty belonged to the hospital where they worked. By and large, the potential ethical issues emerging from this situation were not always obvious so they went without discussion. In the last 20 years, numerous members of the health professions and social scientists have described the roles, role expectations, functions, and status positions of those working in hospitals, as well as the social network within which these workers function. Much has been said about the interpersonal and communication problems that arise, but somewhat less has been said about ethical dilemmas that spin off from organizational, interpersonal, and communication issues.

The male physician historically has had a number of different positions that simultaneously provided him with multiple statuses and freedoms from organizational control; however, he did have a quasi-contractual relationship with the hospital. The sheer power that came from the free movement accorded to the physician within an otherwise formal bureaucracy sharply contrasted with the role of the female nurse, which was profoundly affected by her obligation to represent continuity of time and place. Although the patient care unit was her turf, the nurse and the doctor both knew that in any direct conflict between them they would be subject to unequal privilege within the system. The implicit threat of the doctor's use of the free-flowing communication prerogative traditionally put the nurse in a position of having to use flattery, tact, or even subterfuge in her role of coordinator between the entrepreneur and the bureaucratic system. Many physicians today are employees of health care systems, so the question becomes, How much of the earlier role behaviors have carried over into this new work arrangement or are role relations much the same as before? It is important to remember that the relationship with hospitals has changed for many physicians. A factor that has not changed is that physicians do not remain with patients over a given period of time as do nurses. Nurses are privileged to get to know patients both as patients and as individuals with values, provided they have the time to do so.

In another early essay reflecting the realities of nursing practice but remaining relevant in numerous places today, Esther Lucille Brown discusses the hospital organization as a deterrent to professional nursing. She notes a number of factors including the downward communication of frequent orders, rules, and prescribed procedures issued by persons in authority; the often inadequate channels for upward communication of plans, suggestions, and complaints originating on the lower hierarchic levels of nursing; and the problems of limited lateral communication and psychological isolation can decrease initiative and motivation and encourage dependency, feelings of powerlessness, and dissatisfaction (Brown, 1966). Given what we know of moral distress mentioned earlier, it would seem these factors remain in many hospitals today.

In this era of managed care, diminished fee for service, a nursing shortage, and downsizing, the institutional constraints to good nursing care need to be challenged by the nursing profession. Nursing research needs to more fully examine the differences, if any, that these organizational changes make in the nurse's role and ethics. The presence of advanced nurse practitioners who possess a master's degree and the new Doctorate of Clinical Practice can create a critical mass of nurses with advanced preparation to help all nurses meet the challenge in the clinical role with its ethical obligations.

Nurses traditionally have helped physicians in scientific tasks and also helped overcome inadequacies in the scientific method of practicing medicine. Essentially, the nurse has done this by helping to prevent knowledge concerning ambiguities, uncertainties, and errors from reaching the patient and the family. The nurse has been expected to react with moral passivity to knowledge of hospital events. If nurses had been perceived as full-fledged professional peers of physicians, they would, conceivably, have taken a more active moral stand; however, they have served more as a sponge and a buffer in the system.

Professionals are part of a moral community. They have social links not only to their clients and colleagues in their own profession but also to other groups with whose activities their skills must dovetail. Furthermore, the legitimacy of their professional contribution must be acknowledged by these other groups. By comparison to the professions, semiprofessional groups (which some believe nursing to be) are more bureaucratic and subject to numerous rules governing not just the central work tasks, but also extraneous details of conduct on the job. Semiprofessionals do not have a strong reference group orientation to colleagues and do not tend to see the generalized colleague group as a source of norms. Thus, they tend to be more willing to accept an administrative superior as such a source. One reason given for this pattern in the semiprofessions has been the prevalence of women, who are thought to be more amenable to administrative control than men, less conscious of organizational status, and more submissive in this context than men. Such constraints do not lend themselves to high job satisfaction and can compound already existing ethical dilemmas.

Situations such as the following have become typical due to nursing personnel shortages. On the evening shift in the intensive care unit, where a nurse had responsibility for six patients on ventilators in three separate rooms, the nurse spent about 15 minutes with one patient who was hemorrhaging and then returned to another room to find that a patient had accidentally disconnected himself from the machine, arrested, and died. This incident raised the question of human resources and staff ratios in an area where, by definition, critically ill patients require close attention.

Recent research shows that staffing ratios and the educational level of the nurse make a significant positive difference in patient outcomes (White, 2003). The California Nurses Association used these data and political action to persuade the governor to sign a nurse–patient ratio law that became effective January 1, 2008. This is politics and ethics working together to bring about better, safer patient care.[6]

What obligation do nurses have to voice their concern regarding the ethical or legal aspects of these types of situation? Where would you go with such concerns? Does the state nursing association have a role, and if so, does it play that role to better nursing care through the legal system? Does nursing service leadership have a moral obligation to try to prevent such an occurrence due to staffing problems? One central question has to do with the nature and extent of the professional colleagueship that nurses have with one another and with the nursing service hierarchy. If one nurse raises questions that examine the ethical issues involved in a given situation, whom, if anyone, can he or she rely on for support in the attempt to practice according to the ANA *Code of Ethics for Nurses*? What formal channels need nurses go through in order to have their concerns heard and seriously considered? At the core of these questions lies the larger question of whether nurses have professional, collegial relationships with one another in the workplace and whether such a social network can function to provide an arena in which ethical dilemmas, along with other concerns, can be discussed. As part of this larger question, the role of the nursing leadership must be examined. Given the continuing bureaucratic structure of most health care facilities, what can the nursing leadership in a given facility do to implement the ANA *Code of Ethics for Nurses*? How does this leadership view the obligations and rights of the staff nurse? An important question that has not received sufficient attention is this: To whom does the nurse administrator owe a primary ethical obligation? The person in this role also has multiple ethical obligations.

NURSE–DOCTOR RELATIONS

The doctor–nurse game, first described decades ago, continues to be a factor in daily routines and decision making. One nurse put it this way: "The conflict itself is not so upsetting as the fact that the patient may have to wait hours or a day before the doctor eventually gets around to ordering what the nurse suggested should be done." A lack of effective communication between doctors and nurses can be a significant factor in explaining poor patient care. Nurses have power when it comes to making decisions about their patients, but they must never seem to be giving advice to the doctor. Nurses sometimes pretend they never made diagnoses, although their diagnoses are crucial to the patients' lives (Marsden, 1990).

Nurses sometimes perceive physicians as more deficient in communication and participation-encouraging behavior than in directive behaviors. The desired change in physician leadership patterns appears to require change not only in interprofessional behavior but also throughout the health care system of hospital organization. In the recent past, physicians have not enjoyed a good reputation in their relationships with coworkers. They have tended to regard others as working for them and not for the patient. Despite this delegation of tasks, doctors continue to feel a final medical responsibility, including in ethical and legal aspects, for all that happens to their patients. Have the changes in health care delivery altered relationships between nurses and doctors? Has the increase in the number of women in medicine and men in nursing made any difference in this regard? Would a critical mass of more educated nurses make any difference? Some people say that the ethics world is viewed differently by women and men, while others say the important variable is education (Haidt, 2001).

To fully understand the dynamics of professional relationships among the various groups, it is necessary to realize that in many work settings the nurse is the least educated professional person on the health care team. There are more than 800 Associate Degree in Nursing programs in the United States, and 60 percent of all entry-level graduates have Associate Degree backgrounds (ANA, 2008). While these 2-year graduates are of vital importance to the health of the nation, it must be difficult for them to discuss ethical issues with colleagues with more advanced education. In those situations where each person values the other as important to patient care, such respect can eliminate these potential problems. In the meantime, how can nursing education and nursing service in hospitals help clinical nurses provide better care, including dealing with ethical dilemmas? And what can be done to improve the socio-ethical environment in hospitals? Constraints to ethical nursing are due to multiple factors, one of which can be the medical profession. Another can be nurses themselves.

Historically, the doctor–nurse relationship has been characterized by a fair amount of medical authoritarianism, on the one hand, and nursing's acceptance of subordination or at times deference, on the other. This led to the belief among many nurses that the most fundamental problem in nursing was its status as a woman's occupation in a male-dominated culture. Even the administrative positions in nursing generally were available only with approval of the male-dominated systems in medicine and hospital administration. Historically, the subordination of women and the sex segregation of nursing and medicine helped to establish interactional patterns between the two professions that included subordination of nurses as well as informal doctor–nurse games. Reinforced by hospital training schools and the state laws that restricted the roles of nurses, these patterns led to stereotyped communication and interaction between nurses and physicians, and this in turn was a barrier to the full use of the knowledge and skills of nurses. In nursing, those with ambitions for advancement have historically left the hospital since only by leaving these facilities could they gain any feeling of professional autonomy. Generally speaking, nurses' salaries have improved nationally in part due to the nursing shortage, and so in many places, the issues now are more clinical and ethical rather than monetary rewards and benefits.

Certain practice patterns, such as specialty nurses with advanced degrees, seem to be changing this drain from the bedside. The new, controversial Doctor of Clinical Practice will impact clinical care, and future research will inform us on that impact. In addition, magnet hospitals draw and keep nurses because nurses experience job satisfaction there. The identified elements that drew and retained nurses are in management, professional practice, and education. Essentially, these hospitals are democratic and encourage input from everyone, including in discussions of ethical issues (De Garazia, 2008).[7]

NURSING: A TRADITIONAL FEMALE OCCUPATION

While increasing numbers of men are entering nursing, up from 3.1 percent to 5.6 percent recently, it remains essentially a female occupation.[8] In the past, nursing has drawn into its ranks young women who have had a traditional view of the female role. The picture that emerged was that of conventionally oriented young women who were much more heavily invested in traditional feminine life goals and roles than in career pursuits and reluctant to make more than incidental concessions toward professional involvement. Today, some nurses still view nursing as a job and not as a career or a profession. But for some women in nursing and other professions as well, various factors emerge that make fully enacting a professional role problematic. The work world has been, for the most part, geared to and organized for men and not for women, who often have different and greater family responsibilities. This reminds us too that not only do we often lack good child care facilities, but some men have been socialized to hold certain ideas about themselves and their wives regarding their respective roles both in the home and outside of it. While changes in this regard have occurred, these changes are uneven throughout the country.

Earlier most women who entered nursing had a more traditional view of the female role than other women, especially those in the professions, and this has had serious consequences for nursing and has served to maintain the status quo in role definitions and limitations as well as the decision-making arrangements within hospitals.

More recently, changes have occurred and certainly some workplace environments have become more democratic. Advanced practice roles and many more clinical settings have become available and these changes are likely to increase with the aging of the population coupled with health care economics. More nurses may work in community health or home health than in hospitals in the future as a result of health care reform. These factors along with the general changing view of women in the workforce may assist to further nursing as a profession. However, the fact that now women have more options in the work world than previously, when many women worked in nursing or in teaching, may reduce the pool of applicants in nursing.

As most people know, much reform is needed in U.S. health care. The number of people without health insurance continues to grow. This is costly for individuals as well as for the national economy. A recent issue of the *Hastings Center Report* had a special section "Single Payer Meets Managed Competition," in which after much discussion the position is taken that the single-payer approach appears to be the most cost-effective way to achieve the basic goals of health care (Mill, 1978). Perhaps in the future hospital, nurses and those working in other facilities may practice in a more nurse-friendly environment where nurses can give better patient-centered care and feel good about their work.

The official traditional view of the nursing profession has been that nurses will habitually defend the well-being of the patient as they see it and strive to maintain the standards of the profession. The idea that professional relationships between nurse and doctors and the business model of health care can exert a limiting effect upon the nurses' resourcefulness and, in some cases, increase the hazard to the patient undergoing treatment is exposed. The trust and efficiency that nurses demonstrate are qualities that, in their place, can be of inestimable value to patients, physicians, and hospitals. Obviously, the nursing and medical professions need to find more ways in which these and other traditional roles can be reconciled with nurses' fuller exercise of their intellectual and ethical potentialities. And nurses need to further develop these potentials (Bone, 2002).

PATERNALISM

Before completing this discussion on organizational and social constraints, special notice must be given to the concept of paternalism. In his essay *On Liberty*, Mill wrote that "the sole end for which mankind are warranted, individually or collectively, in interfering with the liberty or action of any of their number, is self-protection. . . . He cannot rightfully be compelled to do or forbear because it will be better for him to do so, because it will make him happier, because, in the opinion of others to do so would be wise, or even right" (Mill, 1978). What Mill essentially says is that we cannot advance the interests of the individual by compulsion, or, if we attempt to do so, the evil involved outweighs the good done. Mill believed that the individual person could best serve as judge and appraiser of (her or) his own welfare, interests, needs, and so forth. Others, including fellow Utilitarians, have vigorously attacked this claim on the grounds that little proof exists to indicate that most adults are well acquainted with their own interests.

Paternalism can be thought of as the use of coercion to achieve a good that is not recognized as such by those individuals for whom the good is intended. Because coercing individuals for their own good denies them their status as an individual entity, Mill strongly objected to paternalism and did so in absolute terms. To be able to choose is a good that is independent of the wisdom of what is chosen, or, as Mill put it, a person's mode of laying out his or her existence is the best, not because it is the best in itself, but because it is his or her own mode. Mill's position has some problems, which remain beyond the scope of this discussion; however, for him paternalism became justified only to preserve a wider range of freedom for the individual in question.

ENDURING ISSUES IN NURSING

The major factor that has caused nurses to leave nursing is undesirable working conditions. Specifically, these undesirable conditions included a lack of administrative support by hospital and nursing service administrators. When conflicts arose between a nurse and a physician, the administrators frequently sided with the physician and did not support nurses. Lack of autonomy, inflexibility of working hours, and being pulled from a familiar unit to be placed temporarily on a short-staffed unit are also indicative of the lack of administrative support. Other difficulties included child and family schedules, frequent overtime with no additional compensation, and in some places, (unjust) salaries. The important factor driving people out of nursing has been the tension of not having a say over their own actions and not having confidence that patients were receiving safe care. The enduring issues voiced among nurses are the following: (a) the status and image of nursing; (b) the effective management of nursing resources including staffing, scheduling, and salary; (c) the relationship among nursing staff, medical staff, and hospital administration; and (d) the maturing of nursing as a self-determining profession (Hanks, 2007).

These conditions that lead to job dissatisfaction for nurses raise many questions about nursing ethics, including the ethics of care, as well as questions about the ethical obligations of nurse administrators mentioned earlier. This chapter has raised questions on the possible organizational and social constraints in hospitals and other facilities that may act to impede the ethical practice of nursing. Several interrelated themes have been developed and include the role and social position of the physician and the nurse in the facility's social system, the bureaucratic nature of that system, the role and power of the nursing leadership in the system, sexism, and paternalism. In addition, the traditional female sex role socialization, which may have been reinforced by some nursing school values, favors passivity in women, including when dealing with ethical dilemmas. In the extreme, it leads to a type of Nazi mentality, where one does a good job by simply following orders no matter the consequences. All of these factors combine to impede change and to make professional nursing practice more difficult.

CAN NURSES BE ETHICAL?

In the first edition of this book, published in 1978, we raised these crucial questions and we believe that they need a reexamination today. The basic question is, Given these factors discussed, can the nurse be ethical? In order to answer this question, other questions need some attention. Do nurses need to become more aware of the ethical, as well as the clinical, aspects of nursing situations? Do they need to think through their own values and ethical stances? What in the workplace can help nurses act on their professional values and ethics? Would a formal mechanism of staff discussion help? Could some structural mechanisms be developed to provide colleagueship within the nursing ranks and between the staff and the leadership levels? Do nurses have a right as well as an obligation to attempt to practice according to the ANA *Code of Ethics for Nurses?*

The concept of caring ethics has been embraced by many nurses. All work that focuses on people takes time and emotional output. How does this emotional work fare under market-driven health care? According to Bone, nurses have developed, sustained, and passed on often "invisible" knowledge and skills with little official recognition. Recent structural changes have diminished the time for emotional work. The nurses she interviewed expressed both anger and sadness over what is being lost (Anderson, 2007).

Nevertheless, we believe that one way to assist in trying to find answers to these questions is to have ways of thinking and a language that is used by many health care professionals in ethical discourse. This book assumes that nurses want to be guided by ethical considerations in their professional activities, and to that end, the chapters have discussed some central ethical dilemmas and nursing practice. To move ethics to a more central place in the clinical setting, it may be helpful to have some ideas of advocacy, formal mechanisms for discussing ethical issues, and the socio-ethical culture needed to foster these activities. A brief discussion of these factors follows.

ADVOCACY

During the 1970s, nursing began an extensive discussion focused on nurses as patient advocates. The ethical responsibility of this role is to see that the patient's rights and interests are protected in health care settings. Advocacy then meant seeing that patients were informed about their rights, provided with facts about their health care situation, and supported in the decisions that they made. This definition of the advocacy role has been further developed and two themes have comingled in these discussions. First, the protection of patients' rights and second, advancement of the nursing profession have come together and in so doing have raised some questions such as the following: Can nurses be assertive enough to take on this role? Do nurses provide organized support for the idea of patient rights and do students learn about advocacy in nursing schools? Do the power structures found in health care facilities hinder nurses from identifying unethical and unsafe practices by instilling a fear of reprisal? If so, are there some facilities that are different? What factors make the difference? (Appiah, 2007; McClure & Hinshaw, 2002).

Several models of advocacy have been developed and the usual one referred to above essentially says that in order for the patient to act as an autonomous moral agent, the nurse also must be more autonomous. All nurses and students preparing to be nurses need to think about this claim that nursing has made. Is it a useful model? Is "the good" for patients contingent on "the good" for nursing? In this advocacy model, (is there) a subtext of whistle blowing. If nurses have the ethical responsibility to protect patients' rights, then they must at times report the incompetent or unethical actions performed by colleagues. This involves possible whistle blowing, which is usually the last resort after trying other avenues to solve the problem.

In the 21st century, with a move toward a national single-payer health system, professional autonomy for all health care professionals may be increasingly limited and more emphasis may be placed on the common good as opposed to the individual patient's autonomy. The challenge is to reach a balance between these two concepts of individual rights and the common good. In addition, nurses may find themselves work-ing more and more outside the traditional settings, which can dramatically change workplace dynamics. Ethical ideals such as patient advocacy and whistle blowing need extensive reexamination and a more sophisticated rendering in the 21st century.

MECHANISMS FOR DISCUSSING DILEMMAS

Ethics rounds can foster the discussion of ethical dilemmas. These rounds are similar to any other nursing or medical rounds, except that the clinical data become background material necessary to examine the ethical dimensions. Health care facilities interested in developing or improving ethics rounds will need to work out the details to fit their particular situation.

Many hospitals and other health facilities have an ethics committee established to deal with those clinical ethical dilemmas that have not been solved at the unit level. From observation of such committees, it is apparent that they function most effectively when a variety of people are members. Professionals such as hospital administrator, lawyer, nurse, physician, hospital chaplain, social worker, and bioethicist, if one is available, together bring a wealth of information and perspectives to the issue at hand. The extent to which an ethics committee will be effective depends on the chair and members, whether the committee itself and others take the committee seriously, and how the committee meets its charge. Such a committee is one obvious place of interac-tion between the ethical and the political. Remember that many aspects of health care are ethical and almost all are political.

In addition to the development of a clinical ethics committee, some institutions have also established a nursing ethics group to address the ethical issues of nursing practice. Such a forum examines ethical problems that relate specifically to nursing and explores ethical choices nurses consider and make on a daily basis.

If your place of work does not have a clinical ethics committee or has one without nursing representation, you and some of your colleagues may want to change that. Also you may find a nursing ethics group a useful arena in which to discuss the nursing ethical dilemmas you confront.

HOW DO WE KNOW RIGHT FROM WRONG?

Scientists in a variety of disciplines internationally are exploring how we reason about right and wrong and have developed a rich body of theoretical work in behavioral economics and evolutionary psychology that examines the rationale behind our ethical thoughts and feelings. Many philosophers argue that doing good, and living a good life, consists of possessing virtues or character traits like kindness, compassion, and honesty and that a good society should aspire to cultivate these virtues in its citizens. But based on the recent international findings from other fields, it is suggested that these enduring character traits, to the extent that they exist at all, may not play much of a role in ethical action. They say that to a very large extent, our behavior is deter-mined by the situation. These research findings have obvious implications for how we think of ethical reasoning and responsibility. Some have concluded that we should place less emphasis on character education and focus more on trying to establish situations and environments where people's better selves can flourish (Appiah, 2007; The Center for Nursing Advocacy, 2008; White, 2003). This conclusion supports recent changes in some nursing work environments.

There has been an attempt to change the socio-cultural environment in hospitals and while controversial, magnet status is one indication that nursing leadership is aware of problems with health care facilities' social environments and the effects they have on nurses. Magnet status, an award given by the American Nurses' Credentialing Center (ANCC), an affiliate of ANA, is given to hospitals that meet the criteria designed to evaluate the quality and strength of their nursing. Magnet hospitals are those in which nursing delivers excellent patient outcomes, where nurses have a high level of job satisfaction, and where the hospital has a low staff nurse turnover rate along with appropriate grievance resolution. Nurses are involved in data collection and decision making in patient care delivery. Nursing leadership values staff nurses and involves them in shaping research-based practice. Nurses are encouraged and rewarded for advancing nursing practice. There is open communication among nurses and between nurses and other health care professionals. In short, a magnet hospital values nurses and has a democratic social environment in which nurses participate in decisions about patients and can be ethical in their practice. In June 2006, the executive director of the Center for Nursing Advocacy presented some ideas as to how to improve hospitals, including ones with magnet status.

Along with the work by professional organizations to improve the social environment of hospitals, research conducted by nurses has made a huge impact. Mentioned earlier, Linda Aiken, a nurse researcher, has presented some of her findings before a U.S. congressional committee (Aiken, 2006, 2007). Other nurse researchers also have had an impact on nursing education, nursing service, and the social environments where nurses practice. It is important to understand that research makes a difference in the lives of both patients and nurses.

To increase nurse participation in policy-making groups, Robert Wood Johnson has developed two programs: (a) Executive Nurse Fellows Program and (b) Pipeline to Placement: Nurse Leaders to the Boardroom.[9] It is also important to know that nursing ethics addresses clinical problems, research issues, and policy decisions.

Questions for Discussion

1. Should the nurse call a physician in the middle of the night about a patient's complaint of severe gastric pain? The nurse thinks the physician will be angry about being awakened.
2. Should the newly graduated nurse refuse to give a drug ordered by the medical chief of service? According to her information, the patient is receiving another drug that may interact with this one and possibly produce negative side effects.
3. Should the staff nurse report the charge nurse for what the staff nurse believes to be an infraction of confidentiality?
4. When a medical mistake is made in the operating room and the patient dies as a result, the family is told the patient died of the disease and that the surgical team did all it could to save the patient. What should the scrub nurse, who was in the sterile field and witnessed the mistake occur, do?

5. The nurse does not like the patient because he is so difficult and acts in such a terrible way to his family and to the hospital staff. She finds it really hard to give him even basic nursing care and just wants to do as little as possible and leave his room. What should the nurse do?

6. The nurse is a member of a collective bargaining unit who has called a strike against the hospital. The nurse disagrees with the union's approach and its issues. What should the nurse do?

7. Does your hospital have magnet status? Should it? If not, how could it improve to obtain it?

8. What does the ANA Code say about nurses' rights?

Notes

1. Bureau of Labor Statistics, www.bls.gov/emp/#outlook

2. Gallup Poll, www.gallup.com/Home.asp

3. Bureau of Labor Statistics, www.bls.gov/emp/#outlook

4. ANA survey 2001, www.nursingworld.org/mainmenucategories/thepracticeofprofessionalnursing/workplace

5. Nursing Ethics, http://intl-online.sagepub.com

6. www.californiaprogressreport.com/2008/01/californians_nur

7. MD–RN collaboration improves work environment, patient care. Anasmartbrief, October 20, 2008.

8. Bureau of Labor Statistics, www.bls.gov/emp/#outlook

9. Robert Wood Johnson Foundation Health Policy, www.rwjf.org/pr/nursing

References

Aikens, C. A. (1937). *Studies in ethics for nurses* (4th ed.). Philadelphia, PA: Saunders.

Aiken, L. (2006). Effects of workplace environment for hospital nurses on patient outcomes. In G. Lobiondo-Wood, & J. Haber (Eds.), *Nursing research: Methods and clinical appraisal for evidence-based practice*. St. Louis, MO: Mosby.

Aiken, L. (2007). Nurse staffing impact on organizational outcomes. In D. Mason, J. Levitt, & M. Chaffee (Eds.), *Policy and politics in nursing and health care* (5th ed.). St. Louis, MO: Elsevier.

American Nurses Association. (2008). National nurses week facts. Retrieved October 27, 2008, from http://www.nursingworld.org.

Anderson, S. L. (2007, August 2). Patient advocacy and whistle blowing in nursing: Help for the helpers. *Nursing Forum, 25*, 5–13. [On line]

Appiah, K. A. (2007). *Experiments in ethics.* Cambridge, MA: Harvard University Press.

Bone, D. (2002). Dilemmas of emotional work in nursing under market-driven health care. *International Journal of Public Sector Management, 15*, 140–150.

Brown, E. L. (1966). Nursing and patient care. In F. Davis (Ed.), *The nursing profession: Five sociological essays* (pp. 176–203). New York: Wiley.

The Center for Nursing Advocacy. (2008). What is magnet status and how's that going? From: http://www.nursingadvocacy.org/faq/magnet.html

D'Antonio, P., Baer, E., Rinker, S., & Lynaugh, J. E. (Eds.). (2006). *Nurses' work: Issues across time and space*. Chicago: Springer Publishing Co.

De Garazia, D. (2008, January–February). Single payer meets managed competition. *The Hastings Center Report, 38*, 23–41.

Haidt, J. (2001). The emotional dog and its rational tail: A social intuitionist approach to moral judgment. *Psychological Reviews, 108*, 814–834.

Hanks, R. C. (2007, October 18). Barriers to nursing advocacy: A concept analysis. *Nursing Forum, 42*, 171–177. London. Blackwell. [On Line].

Horton, K. (2007). The value of nursing: A literature review. *Nursing Ethics, 14*, 716–740.

Jameton, A. (1984). *Nursing practice: The ethical issues*. Upper Saddle River, NJ: Prentice Hall.

Marsden, C. (1990). Ethics of the "doctor-nurse game." *Heart Lung, 19*(4), 422–424.

McAllister, J. B. (1955). *Ethics with special application to the medical and nursing profession* (2nd ed.). Philadelphia, PA: Saunders.

McClure, M. L., & Hinshaw, A. S. (Eds.). (2002). *Magnet hospitals revisited: Attraction and retention of professional nurses*. Washington, DC: American Nurses Publishing.

Mill, J. S. (1978). *On liberty*. Indianapolis, IN: Hackett Publishing.

Moore, D. T. V. (1943). *Principles of ethics* (4th ed.). Philadelphia, PA: Lippincott.

Ratner, T. (Ed.). (2008). *Nurses speak out: Reflections on doctors*. New York: Kaplan Publishing.

Robb, I. H. (1900). *Nursing ethics*. Cleveland: Koeckert.

White, S. V. (2003). Linda Aiken on the health care industry and workplace issues. *Journal of Healthcare Quality, 25*, 21–23.

CHAPTER 5

Rights, Obligations, and Health Care

As nurses seek to meet individual patient needs and to act as patient advocates in health care organizations, they are confronted with organizational goals for cost containment and an acute, worldwide nursing shortage (Buchan & Calman, 2005). One pragmatic dimension of cost containment is that taking patient rights seriously, such as the right to self-determination, gives better patient outcomes while using fewer resources (Summers, 1985). This is, however, a practical and prudential argument for affirming patient rights, not a moral one. The ANA *Code of Ethics for Nurses with Interpretive Statements* (2001) uses the language of rights and enjoins nurses, as a moral obligation, to uphold patient rights. Provision three states that "The nurse promotes, advocates for, and strives to protect the health, safety, and rights of the patient" (American Nurses Association, 2001). The interpretive statements for this provision note that these rights are both legal and moral and specifically include protecting the patient's right to self-determination and right to privacy and confidentiality (ANA, 2001). Nursing considers these rights to be basic rights in health care. While these are important rights in nursing, they represent preeminent values in our individualistically oriented society. But why discuss rights? What is so very important about rights that they deserve separate consideration such that their protection is incorporated into the *Code*?

CONCEPTS OF RIGHTS

The pivotal importance of rights is plainly articulated by Beauchamp and Childress:

> No part of moral vocabulary has done more to protect the legitimate interests of citizens in political states than the language of rights. Predictably, injustice and inhumane treatment occur most frequently in states that fail to recognize human rights in their political rhetoric and documents. As much as any part of moral discourse, rights language crosses international boundaries and

> enters into treaties, international law, and statements by international agencies and associations. Rights thereby become acknowledged as international standards for the treatment of persons. (Beauchamp & Childress, 2001)

The international nature of rights is exemplified in the statements of rights to which many nations subscribe. These include the United Nations' *Universal Declaration of Human Rights*,[1] The World Medical Association's *Declaration of Helsinki on Ethical Principles for Medical Research Involving Human Subjects*,[2] and the *Geneva Conventions* (1st, 2nd, 3rd, and 4th and Protocols 1 & 2).[3] Many other kinds of rights are also affirmed internationally, for example a right to the protection of one's literary or artistic work (i.e., copyright), originally formulated at the behest of the author Victor Hugo in the *Berne Convention for the Protection of Literary and Artistic Work*.[4]

Rights language is widely and fairly loosely used. We hear of a number of alleged rights: a "right to life," the "right to die with dignity," a "right to a healthy environment," a "right to read," a "right to know," a "right to work," a "right to privacy," a "right to clean air" (not to be exposed to second-hand smoke), a "right to own slaves," a "right to bear arms," and many more. But which of these truly are rights, and which are merely hopeful assertions? Where do rights come from? Who has rights? Are there different kinds of rights?

Human rights are the "basic rights and freedoms to which all humans are entitled" (*American Heritage Dictionary*, 2006). Human rights are generally seen as either "natural rights" or alternatively as "God given" that accrue to *all* humanity. Who has rights? All humans have them. The United Nations *Universal Declaration of Human Rights*[5] specifies a number of basic human rights, including both positive rights (a right to . . .) and negative rights (a right to be free from . . .). These include a right to life, liberty, and security of person; a right not to be enslaved, subject to torture or to cruel, inhuman or degrading treatment or punishment; a right to recognition as a person under the law and to equality before the law; to protection from arbitrary arrest, detention, or exile; to fair and impartial judgment under the law, to freedom from arbitrary interference with privacy, and to freedom of movement within the state; a right to a nationality, and more (Universal Declaration of Human Rights, 1948). These rights and more are regarded internationally as fundamental human rights to which all persons have a moral and legal *claim*. That is, human *rights* give rise to legitimate *claims* that can be made upon the state. A general right to protection from arbitrary interference with one's privacy gives rise to a specific claim against the state opening one's mail or a hospital gathering data not related to care. Human rights are incorporated into the civil law of nations: "Human rights are freedoms established by custom or international agreement that impose standards of conduct on all nations. Human rights are distinct from civil liberties, which are freedoms established by the law of a particular state and applied by that state in its own jurisdiction" (Lehman & Phelps, 2004). Legal rights, then, are derived from the state and codified in law.

The Constitution of the United States, the referent for American law, sets forth what people may generally expect from the federal government, its purposes and functions, the relationship with state governments, and what individuals must give up as citizens or residents in order to preserve the collective interests and safety of all. The first 10 amendments to the U.S. *Constitution*, the *Bill of Rights* that was ratified in 1791, set limits upon the powers of the federal government for the protection of the rights of all those within its territories, including citizens, residents, and visitors. While constitutional amendments provide citizens with a very broad array of rights, there is no constitutional amendment specific to a right to health or to health care. Federal and state law, however, use rights language in relation to health. For example, *The Federal Patient Self-Determination Act* confers a right to the use of written advance directives for medical treatment, and individual states grant a right to a minimum of 48-hour maternity stays after normal deliveries.[6]

But where do rights come from and is there a list of rights upon which all agree? Macklin argues that "asserting . . . rights provides no justification for the claim that they exist. Such assertions must be backed up by a general moral theory, or else a sound methodology must be supplied that specifies how anyone . . . can discover the existence of such rights and know what to do when two or more legitimate rights conflict" (Macklin, 1976). Her fundamental argument is that human rights are a matter of moral *decision*, as opposed to *discovery*, and that they can only be ascertained within the context of a broad moral theory, specifically a theory of justice. Any other derivation, she maintains, will result in an arbitrary, ad hoc, list of rights (1976). She mirrors Beauchamp and Childress's position that rights serve a social function to protect persons. She believes that rights language heightens "sensitivity to the needs and suffering of members of humanity outside one's own immediate circle," enhances "the dignity and self-esteem of many people through the official recognition of their presumed rights" (p. 32), "incite[s] people to a certain type of action or to moral reform," and "promote[s] change, . . . move[s] people to action in the form of social and legislative reform" (p. 38).

RIGHTS AND OBLIGATIONS IN HEALTH CARE

Every right has a correlative duty. That is, a right is a *claim* possessed by a particular person that may *obligate* others or the state in certain ways. For each right that an individual possesses, there is a corresponding duty imposed upon another. For example, if there is a right to health care, then there is a duty on the part of another (e.g., the state) to provide health care. More specifically, if patients have a right to safe and skilled nursing care, nurses have an obligation to be knowledgable, skilled, and competent in the care that they give, and further, schools of nursing have an obligation to produce nurses who are knowledgable, skilled, and competent.

A distinction is made between a *right* and a *privilege*. A privilege is a benefit or advantage granted by another. Is health care a right or a privilege? If it is a privilege, no right or claim exists that obligates others to provide care. If, however, health care is a right, then there is an obligation on the part of another (e.g., the federal government or the state) to provide it.[7]

H. L. A. Hart, a British legal scholar of note, identifies two categories of rights: *special* rights and *general* rights. *Special* rights "arise out of special transactions between individuals or out of some special relationship in which they stand to each other" (Hart, 1955). In the case of special rights, the rights and obligations that exist apply only to those within that relationship and not to others beyond it. So the rights and obligations that exist within a nurse–patient relationship, as a "special relationship," apply only to the nurse and the patient and not to the social workers, physicians, or others around them. Those other special relationships have their own rights and obligations. Hart names *promise* as a "special transaction." Another special transaction that Hart identifies that is more directly relevant to clinical practice occurs when one "surrenders rights to another." He writes that rights "may be accorded by a person consenting or authorizing another to interfere in matters which but for this consent or authorization he would be free to determine for himself. If I consent to your taking precautions for my health . . . then you have a right which others have not" (1955, p.184). Hart also identifies natural relationships (e.g., parent–child) as having special rights and obligations. "Co-operating membership" in society, his fourth category of special relationship, establishes political structures of rights and obligations incumbent upon all members of the society (pp. 185–186). *General* rights do not arise from particular relationships or transactions. For Hart, "To assert a general right is to claim in relation to some particular action the equal right of all men to be free in the absence of any of those special conditions which constitute a special right to limit another's freedom . . . unless it is recognized that interference with another's freedom requires a moral justification the notion of a right could have no place in morals" (pp. 188–189). He goes on to discuss the fact that the "general characteristics of the parties ('We are Germans; they are Jews') . . . are not matters of moral right or obligation" (p. 190). That is to say that the personal attributes of an individual do not provide moral grounds for interfering with their liberty. Hart uses the examples of persons who are "improvident, or atheists, or Jews, or Negroes" as attributes that do not allow for interference with their freedom (as did the Holocaust and slavery) (p. 189). For our purposes, it is important to note that age, gender, handicap, socially stigmatized illness, and other patient attributes are not adequate moral justification in themselves for denying these persons the freedom to exercise self-determination and "the right that all men equally have to be free" (p. 188).

Intermediate rights comprise another category of rights. Intermediate rights are specific, material, and adventitious (i.e., extrinsically granted, not inherent or intrinsic) social rights that derive from general rights. For example, where there is a general right to "life, liberty, and the pursuit of happiness,"[8] a part of happiness is found in choosing where to live. The derivative intermediate right is that of owning property where one chooses to live in the realization of one's happiness (Siegan, 2001). Some believe that access to the benefits of health care might fall into this category of intermediate rights.

As critical as rights have been in protecting persons from a range of harms and in conferring freedoms and benefits essential to life, well-being, and dignity, rights-based theories are not complete and full accounts of morality. Beauchamp and Childress rightly note that rights-based accounts of morality "run the risk of truncating or impoverishing our understanding of morality, because rights cannot account for the moral significance of motives, supererogatory actions, virtues, and the like. Such a limited theory would fare poorly under the criteria of comprehensiveness and explanatory and justificatory power" (Beauchamp & Childress, 2001, p. 361).

In addition, framing an issue solely in terms of rights, with no consideration of correlative obligations or responsibilities ultimately leads to a dead end. One can justifiably claim to possess a right even though that claim may not be met by a correlative obligation. This would be regarded as an *unrealized right*. Unrealized rights are claims not recognized as a right by society, such as the claim to a right to health care. If there were a realized right to health care, it would mean that health care organizations and professionals would have an obligation generally to provide care to those in need of care (Gorovitz et al., 1976). This is a general or categorical obligation that does not require that care be given to a person X for whom other conditions may apply. This is to say that not all obligations imply a correlative right. The customary example is that while there is an obligation of charity incumbent upon us all, no particular individual or entity has a right to demand charity of me, absent a special relationship or promise. Beauchamp and Childress affirm a correlativity between rights and obligations but the precise nature of that connection is "untidy" (Beauchamp & Childress, 2001, p. 359).

Nursing has a special relationship with society, and nurses have special relationships with patients that give rise to special rights and special obligations. Few schools of nursing operate independently of all state support. Even private schools receive monies from the state or federal government, such as research and training grants or student scholarships and loans. In addition, patients freely allow themselves to be "guinea pigs" for the nursing students giving their first injection, dressing change, and so on. This "giving" is a "donative element" (May, 1975), a free gift of patient lives to student learning. Thus, schools of nursing partake of the benefits of society as well as preparing students to serve society. This is a part of the larger picture of nursing's obligation to society. Individual nurses also partake of a variety of social subsidies in their education, as well as that donative element of patients "on" whom they learn. The profession, thus, has obligations to society—such as preparing competent practitioners and advancing the knowledge of the discipline; it also has rights, such as having the title "registered nurse" protected by society's laws. Nurses, individually, have an immediate obligation to "give back to society" in competent, skilled, knowledgeable care and a larger obligation in participation in shaping health policy. Nurses also have rights such as to a solid nursing education and to workplace regulations that provide a safe working environment. Nurses also have obligations specific to them and not to others. For example, nurses have an obligation generally to use their knowledge and skills in situations where others might not be present with those skills, such as in assisting injured persons in accidents or natural disasters or in administering emergency basic life support in a public setting such as an airplane.

An assertion of a right to health care necessitates an understanding of what is meant by *health*. In 1948, the World Health Organization (WHO) sought to enlarge the concept of health from an exclusively disease-based focus. WHO declared that "Health is a state of complete physical, mental and social well-being and not merely the absence of disease or infirmity."[9] This understanding of health does make a positive contribution to enlarging health beyond a consideration of the physical aspects alone or disease alone. And yet, it presents a number of problems: (a) it remains rooted in the absence of disease, (b) it is individually focused, (c) it is utopian, and (d) it extends health in such a way as to make it encompass virtually every aspect of life and living. If persons have a right to health understood in this way, do medicine and nursing become entirely responsible for this enlarged "health"? That is, does the scope of medicine and nursing change as the definition of health enlarges? In addition, this understanding of health does not give much direction for development and implementation of organizational and public policies or for meeting the economic burdens that an attempt of this scope would entail for society. It provides no boundaries within which to consider moral or legal obligations to provide health care. Health per se is not always a top social priority, even as the means to other social ends. The concept of a right to health care, particularly this broadly understood, also runs into difficulty when considering that individual choices can profoundly affect one's own health, especially when those choices involve known health risk factors and unhealthy lifestyles or choices.

The 1980s saw a shift from a rights focus (as found in Medicare and Medicaid policies) to a focus on obligations in health care, as illustrated in the important report entitled *Securing Access to Health Care: Report*, issued by the President's Commission for the Study of Ethical Problems in Medicine and Biomedical and Behavioral Research (1983).[10] This Report concludes that society as a whole has an ethical obligation to ensure equitable access to health care. In the Report, *equitable* refers to everyone having access to some level of health care, that is, "enough care to achieve sufficient welfare, opportunity, information, and evidence of interpersonal concern to facilitate a reasonably full and satisfying life."[11] The commission recognized the special importance of health care in relieving suffering and in the social demonstration of mutual empathy and compassion for all citizens. This shift may reflect a renewed concern for interdependence and interconnectedness in community in a society that has emphasized and continues to emphasize individuality and personal autonomy.

The Report asks, "to what extent is the societal responsibility to secure health care for the sick and injured limited by personal responsibility for the need for health care?"[12] The Report concludes that attempting to hold people accountable for behaviors that contribute to ill health has insurmountable problems, including that of discrimination and injustice, as some unhealthy behaviors are more easily monitored or more visible than others.[13] Obesity and smoking are more visible than is the habit of eating foods containing lard. Even some visible unhealthy behaviors may be socially condoned when, for instance, they are a part of "entertainment." Boxing or wild animal acts might be an example of a socially condoned unhealthy behavior. The document *Nursing's Agenda for Health Care Reform* (ANA, 1992) reflects the emphasis shifting from rights alone to personal responsibility. It urges the creation of a health care system that fosters consumer responsibility for personal health and self-care. Thus, a right to health care entails dual obligations: an obligation for the state to provide care and an obligation that the individual bears to participate in attempts to be, remain, or become healthy.

Philosopher Daniel Callahan suggests that the "right to health care" as a social obligation might be undertaken by society in terms of *equal access* to available health care and facilities (Callahan, 1977). While this seems reasonable, such a concept has difficulties because of the competition of health care with other social rights or goods and with other societal needs. A small list of competitors includes publicly supported education, federal/state parks, national defense, infrastructure such as roads and bridges, police/sheriff protection, public libraries, and "greening" the nation. Social goods must be balanced against one another, particularly in times of a troubled economy, and priorities must be established. It is not entirely clear where health care might fall out in a list of national or state budgetary priorities. In terms of an individual obligation as a limit to access, debates still rage as to whether children and elderly persons have the same rights and ought to have equal access to health care, and whether or not those who have lifestyles that put them at risk should have equal access to health care, especially at public expense. Limiting care to those who use recreational drugs, or to smokers, or to those who abuse alcohol, seems reasonable to many; however, the sedentary professor, the butcher who loves well-marbled meats, the well-suntanned individual, or the entertaining stunt daredevil receive a pass. In an era of "evidence-based practice," we have yet to explain *why* individuals have undesirable health habits. Even so, were these data available, it might not influence health policy formulation in addressing questions of responsibility for health and access to care, and perhaps it should not, as the Report of the President's Commission concludes.

There are multiple and often conflicting societal goals for health care. One goal is to contain costs, yet another is to provide equal access to needed care. One possible resolution to the dilemmas involved in rights arguments for health care is embodied in the concept of legislating some form of universal health insurance or a national health plan for the United States. The last effort to legislate a national health security plan in the 1990s during the Clinton administration focused on the language of responsibility rather than of rights, which suggests that today the language of individual rights makes a lesser contribution to the development of public policy that focuses on the common good and recognizes our interdependence in modern society (Bellah, Madsen, Sullivan, Swidler, & Tipton, 1991).

Questions of rights to and obligations in health care are by no means settled. Various efforts are made being made by federal and state governments and health care organizations to control costs and to devise ways to provide health care to the uninsured and underinsured. These efforts at reform give rise to emergent forms of delivery such as "retail" or "convenient care" nursing, with nurse practitioner centers in retail sales environments (Hansen-Turton, Ryan, Miller, Counts, & Nash, 2007; Editors, 2008).[14] An argument could be made that if it is the obligation of both the public and private sectors to assure equitable access to health care, with the federal government as ultimately responsible,[15] then individuals have corresponding obligations and specific responsibilities to consider the influence of lifestyle choices on their personal health and the interests of others. Because we continue to target and label some behaviors as vices (e.g., smoking and obesity), while other vices are not so labeled (e.g., sedentary lifestyle and habitual junk food consumption), we have yet to see how successful this argument or the practicality of enactment would be. As noted above, it is an argument that is resoundingly rejected by the Report of the President's Commission, largely on practical grounds but also on the moral grounds of its potential for discrimination and injustice.

Nonetheless, the availability of and access to medical care must somehow be balanced with considerations of individual responsibility for health promotion and maintenance. That responsibility is customarily framed in terms of a higher cost. The President's Commission held that "even if it is inappropriate to hold people responsible for their health status, it is appropriate to hold them responsible for a fair share of the cost of their own health care."[16]

Arguments about rights to and responsibilities in health care suggest that these debates should give greater attention to such "preconditions" of health as general environmental conditions. Preconditions include clean air, clean water, adequate nutrition, adequate housing, adequate education, and income, all of which contribute to health status (Sparer, 1976). Many of these preconditions (e.g., proper sewage, fresh air, and clean water) were recognized by Florence Nightingale herself. The WHO identifies poverty as one of the chief determinants of poor health (WHO, 2008). In determining the health status of many individuals and communities, these preconditions may be even more significant than building more medical care facilities or developing reimbursement schemes that pay for more medical care. This is an argument for both societal and individual responsibility for health and the environmental conditions, such as poverty, that affect health.

The Report concludes that society has an obligation to provide all citizens with an adequate level of care without excessive burdens.[17] It goes on to state that the costs of achieving equitable access ought to be shared fairly.[18] Efforts to contain rising health care costs, while important, should not focus on limiting access for the least well-served people or the most vulnerable.[19] Taking such a concept seriously means that a state effort such as the 1987/1989 initiative in Oregon to set priorities for Medicaid funding is ethically problematic because it solely impacted the poor who are dependent on public funds for their health care. Efforts to control health care costs that are driving policy development and decision making do impact claims of patient rights to health care and obligations of individuals, health care organizations, and government. As our society struggles to control health care costs and to meet the health care needs of the uninsured or underinsured, we are reminded of Macklin's point that we have difficulty in determining what rights are and how they originate because we have no national consensus on a theory of justice to provide a societal framework in which specific rights are legitimated and can be claimed.

Another challenge remains. That challenge is to determine what constitutes an "adequate level" of health care benefits. This is complicated by claims of "needs" that would have been considered luxuries a generation ago in our society. If one does appeal to needs as a standard for making medical care available, whose definition of needs serves as the criterion? Needs and demands represent two very different concepts in looking at claims of rights to care. Is the health care system obligated to meet insured individuals' demands for use of all available health care technologies even if the medical benefits to be obtained are minimal? How should health care professionals and consumers decide what needs are to be met in providing an adequate level of health care benefits for all in need?

Callahan claims that in order to make such determinations, we must, as a society, determine our goals for health and priorities for health care (Callahan, 1989). He suggests that the first priorities should be activities such as care for the chronically ill with physical or mental health problems and broad public health measures that target prevention and decreasing morbidity. Curing diseases of all individuals and use of all available high-tech care at the end of life would not be top priorities in health care in his view. Instead, there would be an assurance that all individuals would receive needed care and not be abandoned by the community when they need continuing care (Callahan, 1989). The issue of individual patient abandonment has been met, at least in crisis situations, with the Federal legislation *The Federal Emergency Medical Treatment and Active Labor Act (EMTALA)*, which forbids the "dumping" of medically indigent, unstable patients or women in active labor from one hospital emergency room to another due to lack of a source of reimbursement.[20] Such a response still does not address the health care needs of uninsured or inadequately insured persons regardless of the rhetoric about rights to health care.

One way to have enforceable rights to medical care is through a private contract for reimbursement in the form of health insurance. Unfortunately, even if one has health insurance or belongs to a managed care plan such as that offered by a health maintenance organization (HMO), all costs associated with medical care are not covered and often one's choice of provider is limited by an employer's contract with providers. HMOs have achieved varying degrees of success in delivering cost-effective health care. Some have foundered and failed, whereas others are meeting their goals to provide cost-effective, high-quality care to their members, with high levels of patient satisfaction. Unfortunately, some insurance plans such as Medicare still provide incentives for hospitalization rather than ambulatory care or preventive health services. Downsizing of health care organizations and the growth of managed care has lead to patients being discharged from hospitals "quicker and sicker" now than in the past. Because of this, there is an enormous need to develop and finance long-term care and home care services in efforts to provide needed continuity of care that does not simply shift the financial and human energy costs of care to family members and loved ones, most often a female in the family. Cost reduction and cost containment must not be confused with cost shifting.

PATIENT RIGHTS AND OBLIGATIONS IN HEALTH CARE

The overall goals of what has been called the Patients' Rights Movement of the past three decades were concerned with the quality of health care, enhancement of patient decision making, and having some impact on behavior of health care providers to make the system more responsive to patient needs. More specifically, individuals were to be assured a greater degree of self-determination and control over their own bodies when using health care services, which are often characterized by professional and payor dominance, complicated bureaucratic structures and red tape, and authoritarianism. Here, pressures and tensions are visible. What professionals consider to be their obligations to provide care in ways that they feel would be most beneficial to patients are held in tension with patients' rights to self-determination in medical care and treatment, with the added constraints of a managed-care, capitated system. Such systems may sometimes prevent physicians from providing comprehensive information for patient decision making when treatment options are limited to contain costs within the system. Issues of confidentiality, patients' informed consent and decision making, cost reduction or containment, and rationing of health care reflect the conflict that often exists between the respective rights and obligations of consumers and providers (Easley & Allen, 2007).

Another significant issue to be considered in claiming patient rights in health care is the imbalance of power in patient–physician, nurse–patient, or patient–provider–payor relationships. Patients traditionally are in a dependent position that is less powerful, vis-à-vis payers and health care professionals. In most instances, it is still the physician who serves as the gatekeeper in health care systems including access to specialists, although this is changing in some areas of primary care and in managed care systems where nurses often perform a triage function. However, both physicians and triage nurses may also be limited in their choices by payor criteria or protocols. In many of our current health care settings, patients have access to services only with the sanction of both providers and payors.

The patients' rights movement originally sought a new model for provider–patient relationships in which the traditional relationship based on provider beneficence becomes a more cooperative partnership in attaining and maintaining health, a partnership that utilizes a shared decision-making process. The original *AHA Patient's Bill of Rights* (1973), now replaced by *Patient Care Partnership: Understanding Expectations, Rights and Responsibilities* (American Hospital Association, 2003) is demonstrative of that shift. However, the *Patient's Bill of Rights* is presented here in its entirety because it still serves as the basis for patient bills of rights as formulated by hospitals, nursing homes, home care, and other health care organizations. Current patient, resident, or member (as in HMOs) bills of rights generally incorporate responsibilities and obligations as well as rights and are even legislated in some states.

STATEMENT ON A PATIENT'S BILL OF RIGHTS*

1. The patient has the right to considerate and respectful care.

2. The patient has the right to obtain from his physician complete current information concerning his diagnosis, treatment, and prognosis in terms the patient can be reasonably expected to understand. When it is not medically advisable to give such information to the patient, the information should be made available to an appropriate person in his behalf. He has the right to know by name the physician responsible for coordinating his care.

3. The patient has the right to receive from his physician information necessary to give informed consent prior to the start of any procedure and/or treatment. Except in emergencies, such information for informed consent should include but not necessarily be limited to the specific procedure and/or treatment, the medically significant risks involved, and the probable duration of incapacitation. Where medically significant alternatives for care or treatment exist, or when the patient requests information concerning medical alternatives, the patient has the right to such information. The patient also has the right to know the name of the person responsible for the procedures and/or treatment.

4. The patient has the right to refuse treatment to the extent permitted by law, and to be informed of the medical consequences of his action.

5. The patient has the right to every consideration of his privacy concerning his own medical care program. Case discussion, consultation, examination, and treatment are confidential and should be conducted discreetly. Those not directly involved in his care must have the permission of the patient to be present.

6. The patient has the right to expect that all communications and records pertaining to his care should be treated as confidential.

7. The patient has the right to expect that within its capacity a hospital must make reasonable response to the request of a patient for services. The hospital must provide evaluation, service, and/or referral as indicated by the urgency of the case. When medically permissible, a patient may be transferred to another facility only after he has received complete information and explanation concerning the needs for, and the alternatives to, such a transfer. The institution to which the patient is to be transferred must first have accepted the patient for transfer.

8. The patient has the right to obtain information as to any relationship of his hospital to other health care and educational institutions insofar as his care is concerned. The patient has the right to obtain information as to the existence of any professional relationships among individuals, by name, who are treating him.

---

*Reprinted with permission of the American Hospital Association, 840 North Lake Shore Drive, Chicago, Illinois 60611, 1970.

9. The patient has the right to be advised if the hospital proposes to engage in or perform human experimentation affecting his care or treatment. The patient has the right to refuse to participate in such research projects.
10. The patient has the right to expect reasonable continuity of care. He has the right to know in advance what appointment times and physicians are available and where. The patient has the right to expect that the hospital will provide a mechanism whereby he is informed by his physician or a delegate of the physician of the patient's continuing health care requirements following discharge.
11. The patient has the right to examine and receive an explanation of his bill regardless of source of payment.
12. The patient has the right to know what hospital rules and regulations apply to his conduct as a patient.

These rights are legally enforceable only in those states that have entered the *Patients' Bill of Rights* into legislation and where they are already found in the charters of the hospital or agencies concerned. Even if many of these rights are not legally enforceable, they have moral standing and provide patients, families, and providers with a knowledge of rights that consumers might expect and demand as an expression of respect for the dignity of the individual. A declaration of patient rights and responsibilities is even more important in today's health care environment, in which cost-containment efforts so often seem to be driving organizational decision making and recommendations for patient care including, at times, the self-care movement in nursing.

Today, many states have legislated a patient bill of rights, advance directives, and durable power of attorney for health care so that patients' rights and their choices and directions for care do have legal as well as moral standing. The advance directive is an effort to further ensure patients' rights to exercise their freedom to choose or refuse specific treatment when they are no longer able to exercise this freedom themselves. The *Federal Patient Self-Determination Act* (Patient Self-Determination Act, 1995) legislates that patients in health care institutions that receive funds (such as Medicare) must inform patients of their rights to complete advance directives. Patients are not and cannot be required to complete advance directives as a condition of receiving medical care and treatment. Such legislation serves one of the purposes that Macklin points to in her comments that "rights" language and the proclamation of those rights can be used to generate action and appropriate policy development by health care organizations that might not occur otherwise.

The reader may be wondering "why all the discussion about legally enforceable rights?" Are there any rights and obligations that are granted for "humanitarian" or moral reasons based on one's membership in the human community? When attempting to honor patient rights, ethical principles (such as respect for persons, avoiding or preventing harm while benefitting patients, and justice as fairness) and caregiver virtues come into play. As noted previously, rights alone are not an adequate base for a health care ethic.

Some health care organizations have created other mechanisms for taking patient rights more seriously by employing patient representatives. Most often, patient representatives deal with nonnursing and nonmedical matters related to patient comfort and convenience during hospitalization and are more accurately described as management's representative to patients. Attorney George Annas, however, argues that patient advocates should have medical care and treatment as their major concern. In that context, the advocate should have the following powers in order to fulfill the duties of patient advocate: access to all the patient's hospital records; active participation in hospital committees monitoring quality of patient care; power to present patient complaints directly to hospital administrators and the hospital's executive committee; access to all chiefs of service; access to patient support services; and the ability to delay discharges (Annas, 1988). Existing patient advocate systems do not generally follow this model. While Annas agrees that the patient advocates' function is no panacea, it does provide a mechanism for taking patient rights more seriously in health care bureaucracies where paternalistic practices still surface, vulnerable individuals feel intimidated, and physician decisions are often scrutinized for impact on the institution's or managed care plan's "bottom line." Nursing claims to the role of patient advocate may require scrutiny in the light of Annas's recommendations.

FURTHER THOUGHTS FOR NURSING PRACTICE

Nurses claim that they serve as patient advocates. What nurses mean when invoking the term is often not made explicit although *advocacy* is commonly understood to mean identifying and respecting the patients' wishes. This understanding is not entirely appropriate, however. It runs the risk of reducing the nurse to a spokesperson for patient wishes at the expense of the nurse's own moral judgment. Gerald Winslow, a professor of religion, argues that for nurses to serve successfully as patient advocates, there must be (a) further clarification of the meaning of advocacy in nursing practice, (b) a review and revision of states' nurse practice acts, (c) greater public education in order for patients and families to understand the advocacy role of nurses, (d) an understanding by nurses of the difficulties and challenges surrounding the practice of patient advocacy, and (e) preparation of nurses to deal with controversy surrounding advocacy for patients in complex bureaucratic structures (Winslow, 1984). Many nurses are employed in health care organizations in states where patients' rights have no legal standing. One might ask who, then, advocates for patients and their rights to make treatment decisions in what Annas has termed "a human rights wasteland" (Annas, 1988, p. 4). The patient's perspective may well differ from that of the provider; the patient may wish to refuse certain types of recommended treatments or the automatic use of technological intervention when palliative comfort care would be the patient's choice. It has also been pointed out that nurses cannot advocate for patients in the sense of ensuring their rights because nurses are employees. They are not accountable solely to patients even though the *ANA Code of Ethics for Nurses* unequivocally declares, "The nurse's primary commitment is to the patient, whether an individual, family or community" (ANA, 2001). In some instances, patient advocacy by nurses may even incur reprisal. Commitment and accountability are different: Nurses are primarily committed to patients, yet they remain accountable to numerous others such as employers, physicians, and to themselves as moral agents and professionals.

Nurses, in all health care settings, must look at the specific ways in which they encourage or discourage patients' exercise of their rights. As patients or their surrogates expect or demand that patient rights be honored in health care settings, what is nursing's response? Is the individual simply labeled "difficult"? If a patient refuses or does not follow through on a specific regimen because it affects quality of life, is that patient labeled "noncompliant"? How is it that nurses perceive and deal with patients who exercise self-determination, particularly if done vigorously?

In order to fulfill the nursing obligation of patient advocacy, there must be a supportive organizational environment for this kind of practice and a collegial system of nursing care—the domain of organizational ethics. Without such an environment, ethical nursing practice is often compromised by fear and lack of colleague support. Profound changes are required in many health care organizations, including managed care organizations, in order to create environments in which patients can make better-informed decisions and choices related to their health. One way in which patients' goals and values can be considered in circumstances in which they are unable to make their own decisions is for patients to complete advance directives or formally identify a designee for durable power of attorney for health care decisions. There is a growing use of *Physician Orders for Life-Sustaining Treatment* (POLST) forms that are immediately actionable physician orders regarding end-of-life treatments. They do not replace advance directives. Instead, the use of POLST forms is intended to promote effective communication of patient wishes, to document physician orders on a brightly colored form, and to convey a promise by health care professionals to honor the patient's wishes (Hickman, Tolle, Brummel-Smith, & Carley, 2004). The ANA *Code of Ethics for Nurses* and the ANA *Standards for Nursing Practice* can be used to support advocacy for patient care and organizational environments for professional nursing practice. Nurses, as members of a special moral community, can form coalitions and actively work together to create such organizational environments even in a time of restructuring and cost containment (Aroskar, 1995). The integrity of nurses and nursing services as well as patient safety and welfare are at stake.

Other mechanisms to assist nurses in a patient advocacy role include learning to identify situations in which ethical principles and values are at stake; incorporating identified ethical considerations into decision making with and for patients and in policy development and implementation; active participation on multidisciplinary and nursing ethics committees; and initiating and conducting ethics rounds on patient care units. Annas's requirements for patient advocates noted earlier further enrich the concept of advocacy to be considered in order for nurses to adequately fulfill such a role.

Almost 35 years ago, nursing leader Claire Fagin asserted that achievement and exercise of nurses' rights is prerequisite to nurses helping patients to achieve their rights (Fagin, 1975). Nursing's tradition and history have focused on responsibility and service of the nurse as a helping professional rather than on autonomy and the nurses' rights. Fagin sees nurses' rights as emerging from human rights and women's rights, since the majority of nurses are women. One's human rights ought to encompass the creation of situations that will enhance "humanness," for example, feelings of compassion, sympathy, and intelligence. Women's rights involve freedom of choice, equality, and respect for the individual person. This means seeking the right to equal and full participation in such areas as decision making that affects one's practice, the right to influence the environment of nursing practice, just economic rewards, a right to a work environment that minimizes physical and emotional stresses and risk, the right to set standards for excellence in nursing practice, and the right to participate in development of policy that affects nurses and nursing care. One can argue that it is the obligation of professional nursing to exercise such rights. Why? Because, as Fagin notes, the exercise of nurses' rights is prerequisite to nurses effectively helping patients to achieve their own rights.

The assertion of special rights for nurses in their practice is not an end in itself but is the means to improved services for patients and clients and more ethically adequate nursing practice. While the *ANA Code of Ethics for Nurses* (2001) addresses itself primarily to nursing obligations, it also provides a framework for consideration of special rights of nurses derived from the special relationship of nursing to society. Nurses have a right to practice nursing with clinical skill, professional acumen, and moral integrity. When social structures do not affirm nursing's moral autonomy and participation in the clinical community of moral discourse, both nurses and patients suffer. Philosopher Nel Noddings writes that "There can be no greater evil, then, than this: that the moral autonomy of the one caring be so shattered that she acts against her own commitment to care" (Noddings, 2003).

It is possible to argue that if nursing care is considered to be a societal necessity and a right of those in need, then nurses have a corresponding responsibility *and* special right to provide nursing care to clients, care without which clients would suffer. While rights of individuals to nursing care are of great importance, they are not absolute in the sense of overriding all other considerations. For example, patients do not have a right to insist that nurses provide services that violate the bounds of acceptable nursing practice or a nurse's own deeply held moral beliefs, such as providing the means in an assisted suicide at a patient's request.

How do nurses' rights and obligations fit with situations where nurses question whether to accept or to reject care of a particular client or group of clients? Health care professionals have a duty to accept some personal risk of exposure to disease that others are not obligated to undertake. However, it is also morally incumbent upon nurses to minimize risks to themselves by taking precautions that minimize such risk. This is a societal and professional expectation. At the same time, nurses are not morally required to put themselves at serious personal risk from which they cannot be protected, though they (and others) have and may choose to do so. Nurses have the right to the information necessary to make informed decisions about the provision of nursing care in situations that carry personal risk. Nurses may voluntarily put themselves at serious personal risk, but this is understood as above and beyond what can be demanded. Such acts are regarded as *supererogatory.*

Professional standards of nursing practice, the ANA *Code of Ethics for Nurses*, and nursing's social contract with society support the special rights of nursing. It is an obligation of nurses individually and collectively to work together in using these documents and mandates to support their efforts to change inadequate or unsafe conditions of patient care in health care systems. Actualizing nurses' special rights can help patients to exercise their rights and responsibilities. It can also help to reduce financial and other costs of care, such as patient infections, or complications, and injuries to nurses.[21] At times, both nurses and patients may work to improve an institution's care. An early example of patients and nurses exercising their rights together is when nurses worked together in the 1970s to achieve an improved environment for professional practice at the Iowa Veterans Home in Marshalltown, Iowa. The residents became more active collectively in developing mechanisms for participating in decision making that affected their welfare (Maas & Jacox, 1977).

Florence Nightingale argued more than a century ago that a nursing obligation was the development of a healing environment for patients. One can take this a step further to incorporate aspects of a healing environment in any care setting to assure that patients *and* nurses are heard and respected as self-determining individuals, as participants of the community of moral discourse, and as members of the human community.

Nurses must work to ensure patient care environments for the public where standards of practice and the *Code of Ethics for Nurses* are explicitly used to guide nursing practice. Ethical nursing practice seeks to ensure the integrity of nurses and the nursing care received by the public. Securing these, the special rights of nurses, allows them to fulfill their responsibilities and requires a commitment to ethical reflection and to changing organizational culture and policy. In essence, it requires action, often political action. To talk about nurses' and patients' rights without working to make them a reality is to surrender to passivity and continuing dependence on others, or to condone a less than optimal work environment. This is not the needed vision of what professional nursing can and should be for nurses as moral agents or for patient care. Nurses can, do, and should promote and protect patient welfare at the bedside, in homes, schools, and the workplace and nursing rights at policy-making levels of organizations and government.

CASE STUDY I.

The home health nursing department in your hospital is facing budget cuts and staff limitations. In order to accommodate the patients who are being discharged earlier with more acute nursing needs in the home, your manager has proposed limiting visits to some chronic patients. She has proposed closing cases of "noncompliant" patients and patients who show no improvement in spite of visits from the home health nurse for several months.

One such patient is Mrs. Lombardi. She is a 76-year-old woman with a stasis ulcer on her right ankle. You have been visiting her twice a week for the last 7 months, doing dressing changes on the wound and monitoring her diabetes. She has very brittle diabetes, is overweight, and lives alone. The wound is clean but has shown no sign of healing. Mrs. Lombardi is a heavy smoker, with a 55-year history of smoking two packs per day. You have counseled her regularly about the risks of smoking, but she says she has no interest in stopping at this late stage of her life and besides, she has tried many times to quit using many different methods and has never been successful. She is aware that her ability to heal the ulcer may be compromised by continuing to smoke.

Your manager now says that because Mrs. Lombardi continues to smoke, she is noncompliant with her treatment. She recommends, additionally, that you close her case and stop the home visits since the wound shows no evidence of healing.

Further Questions for Discussion

1. Is Mrs. Lombardi acting irresponsibly regarding her health by continuing to smoke?
2. Does she have a right to expect continued treatment given the fact that the ulcer is unhealed?
3. What is your responsibility as her visiting nurse in this situation?

CASE STUDY II.

Mr. Washington is a 68-year-old man with metastatic esophageal cancer. He has been treated for the last 3 years, first with brachiotherapy and later with chemotherapy. The cancer has continued to metastasize in spite of these therapies. He is admitted to the intensive care unit for treatment of pneumonia and placed on a ventilator. After the pneumonia has been successfully treated, however, he is unable to be weaned from the ventilator. Continued tumor growth has completely occluded his airway. The tumor has invaded the brain; he is paralyzed on the right side and shows no sign of recognizing anyone. He withdraws from stimuli, grimaces as if in pain, and tries to pinch or hit the nurses with his left hand. He has developed a seizure disorder requiring heavy medication. Cancerous nodules extrude from his neck, and his left eye and ear have become completely consumed by tumor as has his tongue, which now extends from his mouth about 5 inches and is about 3 inches thick. He receives tube feedings and morphine and fentanyl for pain. His nursing care is quite challenging, and his left hand has to be kept mitted to prevent him from harming the staff. Great care has to be taken to keep his tongue moist and clean. His teeth cut into his tongue and careful oral suctioning frequently results in heavy bleeding from his mouth. The stench from the many tumors is overwhelming and difficult to mask or control. He has been in this situation for 4 months.

His wife, Mildred, holds his Durable Power of Attorney for Health Care and says that he wants everything to be done to keep him alive in any condition. She will not consider withdrawing any therapy and wants very aggressive care continued. Additionally, she demands that his pain medication be kept at a low level so he will be more responsive when she comes to visit. She is very demanding about his care and is loudly and persistently verbally abusive to the staff. The nursing and medical staff are quite concerned about continuing to provide aggressive care. They feel that his existence is filled with suffering and that they are merely prolonging a horrible death. The nurses are particularly concerned as to whether or not his pain is adequately treated. Many nurses refuse to care for him at all, and others have nightmares about torture. They complain that they are being held hostage by his wife's demands for care and fear they are compromising their personal integrity as well as that of the nursing profession.

Further Questions for Discussion

1. Does a patient or patient surrogate have a right to total control over what care will be provided in every instance?
2. Do the nurses have any right to refuse to care for Mr. Washington?
3. Is there any place for consideration of ideals of personal or professional integrity in this type of situation?
4. Must nurses endure verbal abuse?
5. Is there a responsibility to honor a patient's or surrogate's wishes when doing so contributes to suffering and a protracted dying for the patient?

Notes

1. United Nations, Office of the High Commissioner for Human Rights. *Universal Declaration of Human Rights,* adopted by General Assembly resolution 217 A (III) of 10 December 1948. New York: United Nations.
2. The World Medical Association. *Declaration of Helsinki on Ethical Principles for Medical Research Involving Human Subjects, as adopted by the 52nd WMA General Assembly,* Edinburgh, October 2008.
3. International Committee of the Red Cross. First, Second, Third, and Fourth, *Geneva Conventions,* Geneva Switzerland. 1864, 1906, 1949, and 1949 respectively; *Protocols* 1 & 2, 1977.
4. *Berne Convention for the Protection of Literary and Artistic Works,* Berne Switzerland, 1886.
5. United Nations, Office of the High Commissioner for Human Rights. *Universal Declaration of Human Rights,* adopted by General Assembly resolution 217 A (III) of 10 December 1948. New York: United Nations.
6. Congress of the USA. *Patient Self Determination Act of [November 5] 1990* 42 U.S.C. 1395 cc (a) (effective December 1, 1991).
7. W. J. Curran. Notes from lecture given in Human Rights and Health, Harvard School of Public Health, October 5, 1976.
8. Continental Congress. *The United States Declaration of Independence,* July 4, 1776.
9. WHO. *Preamble to the Constitution of the World Health Organization* as adopted by the International Health Conference, New York, 19–22 June, 1946; signed on July 22, 1946 by the representatives of 61 States (Official Records of the World Health Organization, no. 2, p. 100) and entered into force on April 7, 1948.
10. President's Commission for the Study of Ethical Problems in Medicine and Biomedical and Behavioral Research: *Securing Access to Health Care. Volume One: Report.* Washington, DC: U.S. Government Printing Office, 1983.
11. Ibid., p. 20.
12. Ibid., p. 24.
13. Ibid., pp. 24–25.
14. ANA defends the high standard of care advanced practice nurses provide in retail-based clinics. *DNA Reporter,* 2007 November–2008 January, Vol. 32, no. 4, p. 3.
15. President's Commission Report, *Securing Access,* pp. 22–47.
16. Ibid., p. 25.
17. Ibid., p. 4.
18. Ibid., p. 5.
19. Ibid.
20. U.S. Government. *The Emergency Medical Treatment and Active Labor Act (EMTALA).* US Code, 42 USC §1395dd, 1986.
21. American Nurses Association: Written Testimony of the American Nurses Association before the Institute of Medicine Commission on the Adequacy of Nurse Staffing. Washington, DC: American Nurses Association, September 1994.

References

American Hospital Association. (2003). *Patient care partnership: Understanding expectations, rights and responsibilities.* Chicago: AHA.

American Nurses Association. (1992). *Nursing's agenda for health care reform.* Washington, DC: American Nurses Association Publishing.

American Nurses Association. (2001). *The code of ethics for nurses with interpretive statements* (p. 12). Silver Spring, MD: ANA.

Annas, G. J. (1988). *Judging medicine.* Clifton, NJ: Humana.

Aroskar, M. A. (1995). Envisioning nursing as a moral community. *Nursing Outlook, 43*(3), 134–138.

Beauchamp, T., & Childress, J. (2001). *Principles of biomedical ethics* (5th ed., p. 362). New York: Oxford.

Bellah, R. N., Madsen, R., Sullivan, W. M., Swidler, A., & Tipton, S. M. (1991). *The good society*. New York: Vintage Books.

Buchan, J., & Calman, L. (2005). *The global shortage of registered nurses* (pp. 1–26). Geneva: International Council of Nurses.

Callahan, D. (1977, Winter). Health and society: Some ethical imperatives. *Daedalus, 106*, 23–33.

Callahan, D. (1989). *What kind of life?* New York: Simon & Schuster.

Easley, C. E., & Allen, C. E. (2007, October–December). A critical intersection: human rights, public health nursing, and nursing ethics. *Advances in Nursing Science, 30*(4), 367–382.

The Editors. (2006). *The American heritage dictionary of the English language* (4th ed.). Boston: Houghton Mifflin Company.

Editors. (2008, October 15). Retail health clinics provide acute care to patients without a primary care physician. *American Family Physician, 78*(8), 919.

Fagin, C. M. (1975). Nurses' rights. *American Journal of Nursing, 75*(1), 82–85.

Gorovitz, S., Jameton, A. L., Macklin, R., et al. (Eds.) (1976). *Moral problems in medicine* (pp. 426–427). Englewood Cliffs, NJ: Prentice-Hall.

Hansen-Turton, R., Ryan, S., Miller, K., Counts, M., & Nash, D. B. (2007, April). Convenient care clinics: The future of accessible health care. *Disease Management, 10*(2), 61–73.

Hart, H. L. A. (1955, April). Are there any natural rights? *Philosophical Review, 64*(2), 175–191.

Hickman, S. E., Tolle, S. W., Brummel-Smith, K., & Carley, M. M. (2004). Use of the POLST (Physician Orders for Life-Sustaining Treatment) Program in Oregon Nursing Facilities: Beyond Resuscitation Status. *Journal of the American Geriatrics Society, 52*, 1424–1429.

Lehman, J., & Phelps, S. (Eds.). (2004). *West's encyclopedia of American law* (2nd ed.). Florence, KY: Cengage Thomson Gale.

Maas, J., & Jacox, A. K. (1977). *Guidelines for nurse autonomy/patient welfare*. New York: Appleton-Century-Crofts.

Macklin, R. (1976). Moral concerns and appeals to rights and duties. *The Hastings Center Report, 6*(5), 31–38.

May, W. F. (1975, December). Code, covenant, contract, or philanthropy? *Hastings Center Report, 5*(6), 29–38.

Noddings, N. (2003). *Caring: A feminine approach to ethics and moral education* (2nd ed.). Berkeley, CA: University of California Press.

Patient Self-Determination Act. (1995 June 27, Tuesday). *Register*. Vol. 60. No. 123, page 33294 forward.

Siegan, B. H. (2001). *Property Rights: From Magna Carta to the Fourteenth Amendment*. Piscataway, NJ: Transaction Publishers.

Sparer, E. V. (1976). The legal right to health care. *Hastings Cent Report, 6*(5), 39–47.

Summers, J. (1985, Fall). Take patient rights seriously to improve patient care and to lower costs. *Health Care Manage Review, 10*(4), 55–62.

Winslow, G. R. (1984). From loyalty to advocacy: A new metaphor for nursing. *Hastings Cent Report, 14*(3), 32–40.

WHO. (2008). *Determinants of health*. Geneva Switzerland: WHO.

CHAPTER 6

Ethical Principles of Informed Consent

Informed consent is a cornerstone of contemporary health care practice. Because informed consent is grounded in a respect for persons and in the ethical principles of respect for autonomy, it is important to review briefly what is involved in the complex idea of autonomy. Miller discusses the four senses of autonomy used by contemporary philosophers (Miller, 1981). These include *free action, intentional, authenticity, effective deliberation*, and *moral reflection*. Autonomy as *free action* means that a given action is voluntary, that is, not coerced, unduly influenced, forced, or based on deceit or fraud. *Intentional* means that the decision is consciously, deliberately made. Autonomy as *authenticity* means that an action is in keeping with one's beliefs, values, and life plans. Autonomy as *effective deliberation* means that an individual evaluates alternative potential actions and their consequences in the process of actually settling upon a specific course of action. Finally, autonomy in the sense of *moral reflection* means that one acknowledges and acts upon the moral values one holds. These senses of autonomy incorporate autonomy of the will, of choice, and of action. All of these senses are important in bioethics and are actualized through the process of informed consent.

Generally speaking, within bioethics, respect for autonomy means that individuals have the right to relevant information that will inform their decisions to accept or refuse treatments or participation in research. What is at stake here is an *autonomous decision.* The principle that pertains here is the principle of "respect for autonomy" and specifically not a "principle of autonomy." The difference is subtle but of great importance. There is a duty to respect others' autonomous decisions, not a duty to act autonomously. Respect for autonomy means that persons have the right to determine their course of action on the basis of a plan that they have developed for themselves. There is a correlative duty on the part of nurses and the entire health care team to uphold those autonomous decisions. This does not mean that respect for autonomy has no limits. Some individuals cannot make autonomous decisions because they are not *autonomous persons*. For example, very young children, persons subject to threat or other coercive influence, persons with organic brain diseases, persons in a coma, persons under the influence of alcohol, and so forth are not autonomous persons. Decisions that are made based on internal constraints (such as mental ill health) or external constraints (such as coercion) would be called *heteronomous*, not autonomous, decisions.

The reasons people have or give for their actions are their own, but these reasons ought to be morally principled and not arbitrary (Kant, 1964). Even so, arbitrary or non-rational reasons may still be binding. The concept of autonomy, in all its complexities, remains central to the actualization of respect for autonomy through informed consent.

When patients make rationally calculated decisions based on relevant information without undue external influence, they are acting as autonomous agents making an autonomous decision. If respect for autonomy is to have any meaning, health professionals must respect autonomous patient decisions when they do not agree with them as well as when they do. Otherwise, all that respect for autonomy would signify is that we will respect only those patient decisions that we want the patient to make, and when the patient does not make such decisions, we may engage in paternalism, that is, impose our own notion of "benefit" upon the patient over the patient's known strong preferences (Beauchamp & Childress, 2001).

However, the duty to respect autonomy is not absolute. It can be limited if the autonomous action might cause harm. That is, patients are free to make and act upon their decisions and to have those decisions respected, insofar as those decisions and actions do not harm others. Parental autonomy over their children is not absolute either. While there is a presumption that parents will act in the best interests of their children, it is a rebuttable presumption. Some parents have priorities that may conflict with the best interests of a specific child, thus the right to act for their child may be restricted. Another limit to the principle of respect for autonomy and the rule of informed consent is that of emergencies and health crises when patients cannot participate in an informed consent process. In an emergency, if the patient's wishes are unknown and no one can be found to express the patient's desires, health professionals proceed on three bases. The first is a prima facie duty to act in favor of sustaining life. The second is that of a "reasonable person standard" that assumes that the fictional "reasonable person" would authorize emergency treatment. If the patient then recovers and declines further treatment, then treatment is stopped. A third basis is that of implied consent. *Implied consent* may be inferred in circumstances that would lead the team to believe that consent would have been given if the patient were able to do so, for example, the patient requested to be taken to the emergency room prior to becoming unconscious.

While the focus here is on the ethics of informed consent, it must be noted that informed consent has been codified in law. Moral expectations may differ from those of the law. Though there is variation among states in this regard, the standard for informed consent in the law is fundamentally that of *disclosure*. The moral standard, however, looks at decisional capacity; adequate and materially relevant disclosure; patient understanding; voluntariness; and consent. Ethics would also extend participation in informed consent to those whom the law may exclude from the process. For instance, ethics may expect consent to be obtained from children, particularly adolescents, who are capable of understanding their treatment and the ramifications of non-treatment (Kuz, 2006; Roberson, 2007; Tillett, 2005). Under the law, however, such consent or refusal may not be legally effective, and therefore parents may override the youth or adolescent's decision (Community Practitioner, 2005; Tabak & Zvi, 2008).

Guidelines for informed consent, particularly with regard to "status individuals," that is, vulnerable groups, vary by state. It is important that nurses be familiar with federal guidelines and state laws relevant to their clinical population and domain of practice.

Because people can give informed consent only if they have sufficient and adequate information on which to base a decision, an ethical principle guiding the giving of information is veracity, or truth telling. Trust and loyalty in professional relations with clients and patients come in part from veracity and promise keeping and are a part of faithfulness, or fidelity, in relationships. The ethical question is when, if ever, is it ethically justified to withhold the truth as we know it from the patient.

RESEARCH AND INFORMED CONSENT

The doctrine of informed consent arose in response to the horrors of medical experimentation under the Nazis, as they were revealed at the trials of Nuremberg. However, subsequent research that violated moral canons furthered the development of standards for informed consent (Beecher, 1966; Hayes, 2006). Any discussion of informed consent must be placed within the larger context of the moral justification for conducting research using human subjects. In much, if not most, biomedical research with human subjects, we usually assume that preliminary stages or trials have been completed prior to the use of human subjects so that human subjects are never used unnecessarily. Although the moral issues of using animals in research designed ultimately to benefit humans are worthy of our close attention, they remain outside the scope of the present discussion (Crowley & Connors, 1985; Cunningham & Mitchell, 1982; Donnelley, 1995; Donovan, 1990; Nelson, 1992).

In order to proceed with a discussion in this domain, some definitions will be helpful. *Therapy* refers to a class of activity intended specifically to benefit an individual or a member of a group. The person giving therapy has the intention of benefiting the recipient of the activity. *Research*, on the other hand, refers to scientific activity intended to contribute to the general knowledge in a field. Two subtypes of research can be identified. First, scientists conduct *therapeutic research* mainly for the benefit of the subject, while also gaining knowledge. For example, giving a new drug to a cancer patient can be basically for therapeutic purposes and at the same time it can be a trial test for the drug. Second, scientists also engage in *nontherapeutic research* using human subjects to gain new knowledge. An example is an experiment that deliberately introduces change into a given situation and then measures and compares the respective effects on the control group and the experimental group. The control group does not usually benefit in any therapeutic way from the research. The motivation of those participating in the control group is not therapeutic benefit but presumably for the benefit to society or others from the advance of science.

Research using human subjects can and has been justified on both consequentialistic and formalistic grounds. It can be argued that such research serves "the common good" in the advance of medical and nursing science (a consequentialistic argument). In addition, the greater the number of participants in research, the greater is the spread of both the burdens and benefits of research (an argument from distributive justice). The fact that in biomedical research a time arrives when only human subjects can provide the data needed must neither overshadow nor obscure the ethical dilemmas involved.

Morally justifying the use of humans as subjects in experimentation does not resolve all of the possible ethical issues that can confront the researcher once such research gets under way. Such considerations as freedom of choice and coercion, the problem of uncertainty in determining the risk–benefit ratio, rights of the individual and needs of society, and the meaning of "the good" represent some of the more obvious dimensions of these ethical issues. The latter is of special interest because, until recently, biomedical research has largely been thought of as an unquestioned good. Yet, the advance of medical knowledge through research has created both clinical and social problems and is being challenged from many perspectives, including those of nursing (Liaschenko, 1994, 1995; McGrath, 1995), feminist scholars (Holmes & Purdy, 1992; Sherwin, 1992), social critics (Ehrenreich & Ehrenreich, 1990), philosophers (Callahan, 1994; McKenzie, 1990), and physicians (Brody, 1995; Katz, 1993). One important example is from Renee Fox and Judith Swazey, scholars of organ transplantation, who followed the developments in this field from its inception. In a published farewell to the health care community (Fox & Swazey, 1992) the authors poignantly explained that they found the practice of organ transplants to be so troublesome morally that they could no longer chronicle it. Others have noted that when looking at the health care system as a whole, research frequently takes precedence over patient care (Ehrenreich & Ehrenreich, 1990). While these issues may seem far removed from informed consent, they are not, as the history of informed consent is intimately tied to particular social factors in the history of research.

Although the late 19th century saw an acceleration in the systematic use of human subjects for research purposes, this activity did not lead to an exploration of the need for safeguards to protect these individuals. One notable exception can be found in Bernard's 1865 publication, in which he demonstrated the need for research using human subjects and began to develop rules of ethical conduct to govern such research (Bernard, 1927).

Along with medicine, the law gave little attention to the rights of human subjects in experimentation. In the mid-1930s, the Michigan Supreme Court stated that experimentation, although important and necessary, must be undertaken with the knowledge and consent of the patient or someone responsible for him and such procedures must not vary too radically from accepted practice.[1] This broad criterion that the Court used to distinguish between rash experimentation with humans and systematic and ethical scientific research practice could not have anticipated the grave concerns that arose from the Nuremberg disclosures some years later. The atrocities perpetrated by German physicians in the name of clinical research demonstrated to the world the power of medicine for evil. This recognition disturbed many scientists, who then wanted ethical standards, including informed consent, established on a worldwide basis to protect human subjects. There is important scholarship exploring the role of medicine (Lifton, 1986; Proctor, 1988) *and* nursing (Davis, 1992; Steppe, 1991, 1992) in the Third Reich.

REGULATIONS AND HUMAN SUBJECTS

The Nazi experiments on human subjects were inhumane, morally repugnant, and unconscionable. The experiments could not under any circumstances be regarded as within acceptable limits for medical research (Lifton, 1986; Spitz, 2005). The Military Tribunal that tried the Nazi physicians formulated a code of ethics that has shaped the ethos of all subsequent biomedical research. The major contribution of the *Nuremberg*

Code was to make "the voluntary consent of the human subject [is] absolutely essential" (*Trials of War Criminals*, 1949) and inalienable. Furthermore, "the duty and responsibility for ascertaining the quality of the consent rests upon each individual who initiates, directs, or engages in the experiment. This personal duty and responsibility may not be delegated to another with impunity." The *Code* also says that "the experiment should be such as to yield fruitful results for the good of society unprocurable by other methods or means of study and not trivial or unnecessary in nature." Furthermore, "the degree of risk to be taken should never exceed that determined by the humanitarian importance of the problem to be solved by the experiment. During the course of the experiment, the human subject should be at liberty to bring the experiment to an end if he has reached the physical or mental state where continuation seems to him to be impossible." In addition, the scientist "must be prepared to terminate the experiment at any stage, if . . . a continuation of the experiment is likely to result in injury, disability, or death for the subject" (*Trials of War Criminals*, 1949).

The promulgation of other codes of ethics, such as the World Medical Association *Helsinki Declaration of 1964*, the American Medical Association *Ethical Guidelines for Clinical Investigation* of 1966, and the American Nurses Association *Human Rights Guidelines for Nurses in Clinical and Other Research* of 1975, focused attention not only on the ethical dilemmas inherent in research activities but also on the limitation of codes. Succinctly worded and devoid of commentary, codes, although useful as general guidelines, cannot cover every possible eventuality; they are general guidelines that must then be applied to particular situations. These codes of ethics made it clear, however, that the professions recognized that self-regulation by investigators could not be relied upon to safeguard the rights of human subjects in experiments. This realization, coupled with the growing awareness of the limitations of codes, led to the development of procedures to apply the general moral principles contained in the codes.

The procedures took the form of a formal evaluation of research projects by institutional review boards (IRBs) prior to starting data collection. In 1953, the National Institutes of Health developed procedures to regulate research conducted at its clinical center (Faden & Beauchamp, 1986). In 1971, the Department of Health, Education, and Welfare formulated its policy for the protection of human subjects, and at present, these policies vest basic responsibility for the protection of human subjects in IRBs.[2] Because of the prominent role that the federal government has in funding biomedical research, any institution engaged in research must have an IRB. Such institutional boards in universities, hospitals, medical centers, and other research facilities around the country are in charge of initial review of all research proposals and periodic re-review in order to ascertain the scientific merit of the study, that each researcher has outlined the risks and benefits, and that the human subjects have been provided informed consent to participate in the study. Essentially, the IRB must determine that the moral and legal rights and welfare of the subjects are protected, that the risks to an individual are outweighed by the potential benefit to him or her and society, and that informed consent will be obtained by adequate and appropriate methods. These governmental review standards, although worded in general terms, do detail the basic elements of informed consent, thereby drawing attention to its importance.

In spite of these important, substantive attempts to promote the conduct of research in a way that protects human subjects, marked abuses continued. In 1966, Harvard anesthesiologist Henry Beecher published a list of research being conducted in which the advance of medical knowledge outweighed the welfare of the subjects (Beecher, 1966). Many of these studies are now common knowledge and bear an infamous notoriety: the cancer immunology experimentation at the Jewish Chronic Disease Hospital in New York, the hepatitis experiment on mentally retarded children institutionalized at Willowbrook, and the Tuskegee syphilis research on African Americans in Alabama. Although the Tuskegee experiment was initiated in the first half of the century, it continued into the early 1970s, long after the effectiveness of penicillin in treating syphilis had been established. The latter has been explored in detail, including, in the contemporary play *Miz Ever's Boys* (1997), in which physician-playwright Lawrence Feldshul examines the complex relationships between the worlds of scientific medicine, the men, and the African American nurse, Miss Ever, who cared for them.

Although 30 years have elapsed since Beecher's expose, there is evidence that misrepresentation and abuse persist (Alderson, 1995). The fact that proposals must go through IRBs might give the impression that they provide more protection than they do. However, IRBs review research protocols at the local level, and as Annas has noted, "IRBs as currently constituted do not protect research subjects but rather protect the institution and the institution's investigator" (Katz, 1993, p. 38).

An interdisciplinary group, the National Commission for the Protection of Human Subjects of Biomedical and Behavioral Research, was established in 1974 to advise the then Department of Health, Education, and Welfare (HEW). This group was charged to investigate the ethical principles of human experimentation and develop guidelines for the nation. The Commission has published a number of important books that developed from its work. One such book addresses ethical issues surrounding informed consent (Presidents Commission, 1982). In spite of the important contributions of this Commission, an attempt to create a permanent commission for the protection of human subjects failed. Following the Tuskegee scandal, Katz recommended that a National Human Investigation Board be formed, which would have the mandate to monitor, at least, all federally funded research. Senator Edward Kennedy included this in a bill but the bill was never passed. According to Katz, "a major reason why this bill was never enacted may have been the Senate's reluctance to expose to public view the value conflicts inherent in the conduct of research" (Katz, 1993). This shows that the establishment of these commissions and councils and the development of guidelines and regulations are viewed by some professionals as onerous, problematic, or even dangerous, because these activities allegedly may impede scientific advance. Others, however, believe we require even more social control in these matters. They do not believe the present devices, including informed consent, protect human subjects sufficiently from the ever-present potential for abuse at the hands of scientists.

INFORMED CONSENT AND THE RESEARCH SUBJECT

Informed consent should not be reduced to a notion of shared decision making. Informed consent involves an exchange of information based upon which the patient or human subject may elect to participate or refuse to participate. Shared decision making follows upon this choice and involves the patient or subject's approval, authorization, and customarily signature, for intervention or research. The scientist–researcher has an ethical obligation to offer information that includes a detailing of benefits, the warning of risks, and the discussion of quandaries in order to obtain consent from the potential research subject. This consent must be based on the subject's understanding of the information to the greatest extent possible in order for him or her to be sufficiently and adequately informed. The quality of patients' informed consent, that is, their understanding at the completion of the process, should be assessed (Barrett, 2005).

Two early studies that have become classics, published 10 years apart, provide some insights into the ethical dilemmas involved in informed consent. Beecher has been noted earlier, but his work is worthy of further discussion. Beecher maintained that codes of ethics made the bland assumption that meaningful or informed consent was available for the asking, whereas in reality, this very often was not the case (Beecher, 1966). Although he conceded that consent in the fullest sense may not be obtainable, he said that it remains a goal toward which every researcher must nevertheless strive. With this in mind, he reviewed 50 studies, out of which only 2 mentioned informed consent; 12 studies seemed outright morally repugnant; generally his data suggested widespread ethical issues, especially with regard to informed consent. Following the position of the British Medical Research Council, Beecher said that not only should all investigations be conducted in an ethically right-making manner, but in the publications, it should also be made unmistakably clear that moral strictures have been observed. He believed that journals have a moral obligation not to publish unethical research, even when those studies present very valuable data. Beecher believed that such a policy would discourage unethical experimentation. It is interesting to note that there has been discussion in the public domain about the ethical implications of using the data obtained through Nazi experimentation (Beecher, 1966; Caplan, 1989; Seidelman, 1989). Beecher concluded by pointing out that an ethically acceptable approach has two important components: informed consent and the presence of an intelligent, informed, conscientious, compassionate, and responsible investigator.

The other landmark study, by Barber, published in 1976, made note of the fact that in the previous decade, we had increasingly perceived a social problem in the abuse of human subjects in medical experimentation (Barber, 1976). Experimentation utilizing human subjects was of concern on two counts: (a) the increased power, scope, and funding of biomedical research and (b) changes in values that have increased the emphasis on equality, participation, and the challenging of arbitrary authority. Barber and his colleagues conducted a brief survey in which they found investigators who were "permissive" regarding both informed consent and the risk–benefit ratio they were willing to accept. These data raise the question of how it happens that the treatment of human subjects is sometimes less than morally right-making, even in some of the most respected university hospitals. Barber answered this question by saying that these abuses can be traced to defects in the training of researchers, to defects in the screening and monitoring of research by review committees, and to a fundamental tension between investigation and therapy. Katz (1993) notes that defects in training have been corrected and that IRBs have generally become stronger. However, there remains a tension between research and therapy, which may be internal to the practice of scientific medicine. This will be discussed further momentarily.

In another early study, Gray interviewed 51 women who were, or had just been, subjects in another study to determine the effects of a new labor-inducing drug. His findings indicated that although all 51 women signed a consent form, 20 of them learned only from Gray's interview that they were research subjects. Of this group of 20, most of them did not understand that there might be hazards, that they would be subjected to special procedures, or that they were not required to participate in the study. Indeed, four of the women made it clear that they would not have participated had they understood and realized that they had a choice (Gray, 1975). This points to an important aspect still relevant today: a signed form does not necessarily mean that *informed* consent has been obtained (McMullen & Philipsen, 1993). As Curtin indicates, "although the legal doctrine of informed consent arose to protect patients, the consent form arose to protect providers" (Curtin, 1993, p. 18).

For many, the core of the informed consent process has been the balancing of risk to the human subject against possible benefits to the individual and society. However, Jonas, an early critic of this conception, voiced resistance to this "merely utilitarian view." He raised the issue of the peculiarity of human experimentation quite independent of the question of possible injury to the subject. Jonas argues that the wrong entailed in making a person an experimental subject is not so much that the person is made a means to an end, since that happens in social contexts of all kinds, but rather that the person is made a "thing." He asserts that this approach reduces the human subject to a human object, to a passive thing or token, or a "sample" merely to be acted upon (Jonas, 1969, pp. 1–31). It is a potent critique that merits attention in research design and implementation.

Informed consent necessitates truth telling on the part of the researcher and free and informed choice on the part of the subject within a context of some degree of uncertainty. If all possible risks and benefits of a given procedure or drug were known, the research would be unnecessary. *The Declaration of Helsinki*, initially promulgated in 1964 (sixth revision in 2008), states that research involving human subjects cannot legitimately be carried out unless the importance of the objective is in proportion to the inherent risk to the subject. Such inherent risks may be easier to measure and weigh in the risk–benefit calculus with biomedical research than with research focused on psychological or social aspects. Nevertheless, *The Declaration of Helsinki* does say that every precaution should be taken to minimize the impact of the study on the subject's physical and mental integrity and on the personality of the subject.[3]

It has been documented that the social sciences differ from the natural sciences in some fundamental ways. "Qualitative research" is the generic descriptive term for social science research that does not model the natural sciences but rather seeks to understand a given phenomenon from the perspectives of the subjects. Increasingly utilized in nursing, qualitative research has been conducted to a great deal by anthropologists and sociologists. In contrast to biomedical research, qualitative research does not involve invasive bodily procedures, and because the data are produced by conversation, this research implies a different relationship between the investigator and the research participant. Nonetheless, there are several ethical issues involving protection of research participants (Holloway & Wheeler, 1995). Central among these are issues of deception (mentioned below), trust, and confidentiality (Haggerty & Hawkins, 2000). Confidentiality is particularly important because the participants could be easily identified. Given the often sensitive nature of the topics under study, there could be grave consequences to participants if confidentiality were breached.

How much disclosure is necessary for informed consent to be a possibility? Entry into the hospital is no longer regarded as "blanket consent" to treatment. Today the "volume" of information is much less important than the quality and relevance of disclosure. The emphasis has shifted from what the physician discloses to what the patient understands. That is, the emphasis has shifted from a professional standard of practice to a concern for patient rights and autonomy.

Nearly 50 years ago, sociologist Parsons noted that patients are made vulnerable by sick-role helplessness, a lack of technical competence, and the emotional disturbance experienced in the sick role. The patient is, thus, ripe for exploitation (Brody, 1992). Parsons points to inequalities of knowledge and power between the professional who obtains informed consent and the patient who grants it (Parsons, 1951). This power differential has been of substantial concern to feminist and post-colonial theorists. This power differential, coupled with sick-role vulnerability (even if today not as passive as had been described by Parsons in the 1950s), and historic and enduring failures at researcher self-policing make informed consent acutely necessary.

In early discussions of informed consent, Baumrind made one of the more profound observations regarding human experimentation. She maintains that subjects are less adversely affected by physical pain or psychological stress than by experiences that result in loss of trust in themselves and the investigators and, by extension, in the meaningfulness of life itself. Researchers violate the fundamental moral principles of reciprocity and justice when their acts deceive or degrade those whose trust has been extended to them. The harm that is done accrues both to the individual subject and to society (Baumrind, 1973). It is worth noting that within contemporary society, there is widespread mistrust of experts, that is, those with special knowledge such as physicians, attorneys, business leaders, scientists, and to a lesser extent, academics. Historically, these groups have been granted enormous social privilege, including the pursuit of self-interest, precisely because they have been charged with and thought to be serving a larger, social good. In recent history, medicine has engaged in research that relied upon deception to obtain its findings (Hofling et al., 1966; Humphreys, 1970; Rosenhan, 1973). Progress has been made: none of these studies would, today, pass muster with an IRB. The question is usually raised as to whether this means that some research cannot or should not be performed. Yes, it does possibly mean just that. Although we have been concerned with deception in the practice of research, it is not limited to research. Deception can be used for the ostensible good of reassuring patients (Teasdale & Kent, 1995). But trust is always violated when deception is used. Deception is ethically unacceptable.

Sometimes research findings can be biased if too much information is given to the potential subject. In such cases, at least two solutions to the issue of informed consent exist. First, it may be possible to redesign the research so that disclosure will not bias the study. Second, it may be possible to tell the subject that some details will be withheld to preserve the validity of the findings. Consent is then sought from a subject who knows that specific details are being withheld. The caveat here is that the information that is not disclosed must not be materially relevant to the patient's decision to participate and must not increase the subject's risk of harm.

While the actual practice is imperfect, the process of informed consent treats subjects as persons rather than as objects. Insofar as every treatment procedure and every involvement in research carry with them potential risk, it must be the patient or his or her guardian who has the right to decide not only whether to participate but also what factors are or are not relevant to his or her consent.

INFORMED CONSENT AND SELECTED HUMAN SUBJECTS

The concept of informed consent rests on the assumption that the researcher will adequately inform the potential research subject. To do so, information must be communicated in language that the patient can comprehend, so that the risks and benefits are well understood (Cohn & Larsen, 2007). Only then will a patient be in a position either to agree to participate or to refuse to do so. The language of the patient refers not only to the language the patient speaks, whether Spanish, English, or any other language, but also to the educational level of discourse, as well as to language that is common. Strides have been made to improve written consent forms, by reframing "medicalese" and "legalese" in common language (Lorenzen, Melby, & Earles, 2008). Refusal to participate must not negatively affect the relationship with the researcher or the institution providing the service.

Persons with *decisional capacity* have the right to decide for themselves whether to accept or reject proposed treatment, including participation in a research protocol. *Competence* is a legal designation and is not a clinical judgment made by health care professionals. Legally, persons are presumed to be competent unless declared otherwise by the courts. A person with decisional capacity has the ability to communicate choices, can understand relevant information, can appreciate the situation and its consequences, and can manipulate information rationally (Appelbaum & Grisso, 1988; Erlen, 1994a, 1994b, 1995; Silva, 1993). Other work on decisional capacity and competence adds the important dimension of making decisions in keeping with one's values or how one lives life (White, 1994). Certain groups present special ethical issues and raise questions regarding the adequacy of informed consent. Research using "status individuals," that is, persons who fall within a vulnerable category (e.g., students, prisoners, minors, those who are mentally ill or developmentally delayed, elderly persons, especially those persons in an institution, and fetuses), raises somewhat different issues.

The problem of "restricted choice" is a central concern in discussions of informed consent. Restricted choice raises the question of moral limitations to consent in situations or settings where choices are limited. Students are subject to faculty in ways that restrict their choices, such as a decision not to participate in faculty research. Prisoners exist within institutional settings that restrict both their environment and their choices. Offering payment for participation in such settings may be unduly influential.

Similar issues arise in research with the committed mentally ill patient. Voluntarily institutionalized patients may be adequately protected by the process of informed consent. Patients whose mental status led to involuntarily institutionalization may be unable to give informed consent. Laws in some states have addressed the informed consent issue for both involuntary and voluntary patients with regard to the right to refuse drugs. However, the question has been raised as to whether such legislation really provides a useful safeguard for the protection of the psychiatric patient's civil rights. With persons who are cognitively impaired or developmentally delayed, the problems are twofold: the individual's intrinsically diminished capacity and the extrinsic influence of institutionalization and dependency. Diminished capacity is not necessarily no capacity and attempts should be made to assess rather than assume the level of the person's capacity (Grebe, 2007; Nokes & Nwakeze, 2007; Slaughter, Cole, Jennings, & Reamer, 2007).

Some of the same kinds of issues come into play in research with minors (Broome & Stieglitz, 1992; Fowler, 1988; Thurber, Deatrick, & Grey, 1992). One of the most serious questions with any group—and especially vulnerable ones, including healthy children—involves research that is nontherapeutic or nonbeneficial to the subject. On what ethical grounds should research be conducted using either healthy children or mentally ill or retarded children where risks must be weighed against benefits? For normal children, the benefits will be neither direct nor immediate in any tangible way. The following questions arise: Should physically well, normal children ever be human subjects? If so, on what moral grounds? Should mentally ill or retarded children participate in any research, and, if so, should it only be research that can potentially benefit them directly? If other research is to be permitted, on what moral grounds would these children become human subjects and who will speak for them in the informed consent procedure?

Research on fetuses raises issues of possible medical benefits gained as measured against the possible ethical costs of such research to society. Some of this impassioned debate surrounding fetal research is tied to the different moral positions that people have taken on abortion. A federal ban on fetal research initiated in 1988 was subsequently lifted in response to the arguments that many diseases and possible treatments could be explored through research on fetuses (Markowitz, 1993; Sanders, Giudice, & Raffin, 1993; Shorr, 1994). Seemingly irreconcilable debate still rages over the uses of fetuses as research subjects.

Older adults, and particularly those in institutions such as nursing homes, represent another vulnerable group in the human subjects controversy (Butterworth, 2005). Because cognitive functioning is more frequently impaired in elderly persons than in other adults, decisional capacity is of particular concern (Alt-White, 1995). And, as with some of the other status groups noted above, there are socially negative views of the group that obscure some of the ethical considerations.

Despite its monumental importance, informed consent alone is not adequate to protect patients (Grace & McLaughlin, 2005). The attitude of the researchers themselves is as important as the informedness of potential subjects. Katz argues that it is imperative that researchers be committed to the *idea* of informed consent (Katz, 1993). Such a commitment would serve to keep at bay the powerful pull to advance medical knowledge at any cost over the welfare of those human subjects who participate in the research that advances medical knowledge.

INFORMED CONSENT AND TREATMENT

The elements of informed consent operative in research are also pertinent to treatment choices (Aveyard, 2005). Patients should not receive treatment, except in emergencies, until they have given consent that is informed. In treatment, we assume that patients benefit directly, whereas in research, they may or may not benefit directly in return for participation. And yet, the boundaries between treatment and research are often less distinct, particularly with certain diseases.

The introduction of what has come to be called *compassionate use protocols* demonstrates this blurring of boundaries. Compassionate use protocols are research protocols designed to test interventions on human subjects that have not been proven but may be helpful in treating a specific disease, for example, cancer or AIDS. Compassionate use protocols may be justified because the known risk of mortality is seen as sufficient to balance the unknown risks that might be associated with possible benefit. It cannot be assumed that someone with a fatal disease for which there is no cure would automatically desire to participate in a compassionate use protocol. At the same time, it should be noted that patient groups, particularly those with AIDS and breast cancer, have been very active in lobbying for earlier access to potential (as yet unapproved) therapies. In these situations, as in all clinical situations, it is important that patients receive honest and detailed information about the interventions that are available and how those interventions may profoundly affect their lives.

It was not always commonplace for physicians to tell patients their diagnosis and prognosis, especially if it were a tragic prognosis. Uniform disclosure of diagnosis and prognosis has become part of the mainstream culture of American medicine since the rise of consumerist movements in the 1960s and 1970s. It was in this period that medical paternalism came under closer scrutiny and general disapproval. The reasoning underlying the decision to withhold information went something like this: "The patient is very ill and is suffering. We should not further burden him or her with knowledge of the seriousness of the diagnosis. It will do more harm than good." Such good intentions in the name of doing no harm result in the curtailment of the patient's autonomy and create a deceitful situation for all those around the patient. As concern for patient rights and respect for patient autonomy escalated, withholding of information and medical paternalism in general came to be seen as morally unacceptable. The pendulum swung perhaps too far in the other direction, and information, actually an overabundance of information, came to be all but imposed upon patients.

Unique challenges to the view that "all patients must be informed" are presented by persons from differing cultures where decision making is left more explicitly to medical authority or is more communal than we customarily understand it to be (Blackhall, Murphy, Frank, Michel, & Azen, 1995; Carrese & Rhodes, 1995; Orona, Koenig, & Davis, 1994; Shaibu, 2007). A research project on ethical decision making in end-of-life decisions among Chinese-Americans, Hispanic-Americans, African-Americans, and Anglo-Americans demonstrated cultural differences in understanding regarding informing patients (Davis & Koenig, 1996; Koenig & Marshall, 1994). Because informed consent exists, in principle, to honor and respect a person's autonomy, differences in cultural understanding of autonomy (e.g., as family autonomy) and informedness should be studied (Mathar & Morville, 2006; Pérez & Borbolla, 2007).

How information is conveyed is related to whether informed consent is conceived of as an event or a process. As an event, informed consent is seen as occurring in a single time period, whereas as a process, informed consent takes place over time (Wear, 1993). In the complex reality of practice, these are not mutually exclusive, and process strategies such as anticipatory guidance may be utilized to prepare patients or families for the consent event (Yamokoski, Hazen, & Kodish, 2008).

Another contemporary issue regarding informed consent and treatment concerns managed care and the disclosure of treatment availability. In the move to managed care, insurance companies increasingly dictate what treatments will and will not be paid for. These policies, however, are not routinely made available to patients and this raises questions as to the ethical obligation that these institutions have to those for whom they are responsible for the provision of care. Several works address these issues and others related to managed care (Council on Ethical and Judicial Affairs, 1995; Menzel, 1990; Morreim, 1995a, 1995b; Reiser, 1994; Rodwin, 1993, 1995).

Informed consent is not a perfect tool, but with more attention to the ethics underlying it and a focus on the pragmatic aspects of the process, the patient should be better able to participate in the decision making involved in his or her treatment and care.

INFORMED CONSENT AND NURSING

Over the past 30 years, the discipline of nursing has continued to address ethical issues in nursing practice and research. The following is a brief overview of selected aspects of informed consent in research and treatment and the nurse's obligations as presented in those writings. Abdellah, in a paper based on a presentation at the 1967 National League for Nursing Convention, noted that as nursing research focuses more on clinical problems, the legal and ethical aspects will become more apparent. Although clinical nursing research may differ from medical research in the extent and kind of risk to patients, in both disciplines many similar problems exist regarding the conduct of research (Abdellah, 1967).

In the mid-1960s, nurse investigators were just beginning to make inroads in biological research. At that time, the nature of consent to participate in research as a human subject could be implicit, explicit, implied, or in the form of a written statement. The fact that a patient was admitted to a hospital "implied" consent to treatment. Recall that Beecher's paper chronicling research abuses was published in 1966. With the advent of governmental guidelines for the use of human subjects and the establishment of peer review committees to assist in safeguarding the rights of human subjects through a formal informed consent procedure, the informal and blanket mechanisms, which could be too easily abused, were set aside.

In 1969, Berthold wrote a detailed paper based on a review of the literature and focused on the larger topic of maintaining human rights and values amidst a scientific-technological revolution and the concomitant social revolution. She developed the idea that the right of the individual in American society to dignity, self-respect, and freedom of self-determination has been in conflict with the rights and long-range interests of society on many occasions and on various issues. Berthold went on to say that these conflicts have generally been characterized as involving humanitarian, libertarian, and scientific values. Humanitarian values have to do with respect for the sanctity of human life and the safeguards needed to protect the subject from physical or emotional harm. Libertarian values have to do with the individual's political, civil, and individual rights to self-respect, dignity, freedom of thought and action, and the safeguards needed to protect the individual from invasion of privacy without his or her knowledge for the sake of the research itself. Scientific values concern the safeguards needed to protect the right to know anything that may be known or discovered about any part of the universe. In specific situations, these different values lead to competing moral claims that had to be balanced against one another within the process of moral reasoning (Berthold, 1969).

Today, we might wonder if this value of the right to know anything has contributed to a scientific totalitarianism (Liaschenko, 1994, 1995). Might not this cultural value be responsible at least in part for some of the abuses committed in the name of the advance of medical knowledge? Evidence of this is given in the argument published in 1977 by a nurse and a physician working in a burn center (Imbus &

Zawacki, 1977). They argued that in burn cases where survival is unprecedented, the person should be allowed to die. The answer by the National Institutes of Health (NIH) consensus conference on the treatment of burns was that people must always be treated because to do otherwise would impede research (Schwartz, 1979). Informed consent would, thus, be rendered irrelevant in such a situation—the patient would not be permitted to refuse treatment.

Scientific inquiry can involve several specific ethical issues, all of which should be considered by the nurse investigator when designing research as well as by the potential human subject giving informed consent. These issues include (a) loss of dignity and autonomy, (b) invasion of privacy, (c) time and energy requirements, (d) mental and physical discomfort or pain, and (e) risk of physical or emotional injury. These issues must be weighed against potential benefits for the subject personally, for people with similar conditions (e.g., diabetics), and for the general good of all people. Although respect for autonomy has been increasingly questioned as a basis for practice, it is essential if the demand for the advance of medical knowledge is not to trump individual patient wishes.

In 1970, Batey raised the question as to when and to what extent the issue of the rights of human subjects becomes a methodological issue in nursing research. She also asked whether there is a metaprofessional ethic or a set of values guiding nurse researchers who are both researchers and clinicians. In addition, she asked whether nurse researchers share a set of values directed toward optimizing the conditions needed for fulfillment of the aims of science (Batey, 1970).

The American Nurses Association (ANA) has been active in developing guidelines on ethical values for the nurse in research. In 1968, the Committee on Research and Studies said that nursing was committed to the identification and elaboration of a body of scientific knowledge that guides nursing practice in the provision of optimal nursing services to society. The ANA reaffirmed its belief in the rights and the responsibilities of members of the profession to conduct research and to meet its obligations to those members by establishing guidelines on ethical values. In discussing these ethical dimensions within the framework of protecting human rights, the ANA elaborated on the rights to privacy, to self-determination, to conservation of personal resources, to freedom from arbitrary hurt, and to freedom from intrinsic risk of injury. The rights of minors and persons lacking decisional capacity, such as young children or unconscious patients, and the informed consent process were also discussed. Essentially, the ANA's position rests on the idea that the relationship of trust between subject and investigator requires that the subject be assured that he or she will be treated fairly and that no discomfort, risk, or inconvenience, beyond that initially stated in obtaining informed consent, will be imposed without further permission being obtained from the subject (American Nurses Association Committee on Research and Studies, 1968).

The nurse who conducts research does not differ from colleagues in other disciplines. The proposed research must have scientific merit and meet the quality standards of the sciences or humanities. The ANA *Code of Ethics for Nurses with Interpretive Statements* (2001) states that the researcher must be qualified to conduct the specific research proposed. The research proposal must be reviewed by a qualified review board that will ensure patient protection and the ethical integrity of the research (ANA, 1968). Then, the research protocol and activities must ensure that the human subject will be informed in understandable language and will in no way be coerced to participate or continue in the study but will be free to exercise his or her freedom to refuse or cease participation. Personal integrity and ethical understanding of the investigator are essential to preserve the safety and the rights of the human subject. Nursing must continue its discussions within the profession of the issues involved in research with human subjects, informed consent, and the conflicting moral claims that create ethical dilemmas for the nurse researcher who is the principle investigator and for the nurse in the clinical setting who assists in another's research.

The ethical issues that might arise for nurses who assist in another's research received official attention in the 1975 ANA position paper on human rights developed by the Commission on Nursing Research. One very important aspect of this document is its statement on human rights for the nurse (American Nurses Association Commission on Nursing Research, 1975).

> Implementation of this guideline implies the need for written statements about conditions of employment and any special expectations about work performance above and beyond that customarily expected of a nurse. In advance of employment, nurses need to know if they will be expected to provide medicine, treatment, and other procedures as part of double-blind investigations. They need to know in advance if the work requires them to function as data collectors for research in addition to their role as nurses engaged in the direct delivery of patient care services. Conditions of employment must also provide for the option of not participating in clinical research if these work expectations are not spelled out in advance of employment.*

Little is known about the ethical experiences of nurses who participate in research data collection for others. Nurses, however, bear an instrumental relationship to the ends of medicine; that is, in carrying out orders they become the means to the therapeutic ends set by others, usually physicians. Although not specifically looking at nurses conducting research, in a study examining the ethical concerns of nurses, Liaschenko demonstrates that nurses are harmed when they must carry out treatment which they consider destructive (Liaschenko, 1995). They are harmed because they experience moral distress (American Nurses Association Committee on Research and Studies, 1968) and they are harmed because the integrity of their practice is violated.

Another important group about which we know little is the nurses who run clinical trials. So far the discussion has focused on nurses conducting nursing research. Yet it is primarily nurses who run the clinical trials of medical research and who obtain consent—and who need particularized information about consent in clinical trials (Cantini & Ells, 2007). These nurses are paid by research money, hired by physicians, and are responsible to them. Serious concerns about informed consent are not uncommon. These nurses potentially face very difficult ethical dilemmas around issues of responsibility and conflict of loyalty. The world of practice is not neat and tidy and living by one's commitments can be difficult. Most of us make compromises and indeed, doing so wisely and with integrity can be ethically appropriate (Winslow & Winslow, 1991).

---

*Reprinted with permission of the American Nurses Association.

Silva identifies nine principles essential to the ethical conduct of research. These include:

1. Respect for the autonomous person to consent
2. The prevention of harm and the promotion of good
3. Respect for personhood and the valuation of diversity
4. Respect of benefits and burdens of research in terms of the selection of subjects
5. Protection of privacy
6. Maintenance of the integrity of the researcher
7. Reporting of scientific misconduct
8. Maintenance of the investigator's competence
9. A concern for animal welfare, if they must be used (Silva, 1995a)

These principles and the commentary that accompanies them provide a framework for critical ethical reflection in nursing research (Silva, 1995b).

Informed consent was explored in detail in the first book on ethics and nursing research, *Patients, Nurses, Ethics,* by Davis and Krueger (1980). As we have seen, it continues to figure centrally in the literature on nursing ethics whether in relation to research or treatment. Although most of this recent work is not data based, it does support earlier studies showing the concerns of nursing in informed consent (Davis, 1988, 1989a, 1989b). For example, one of these studies identified five roles in which nurses have assumed active involvement in informed consent. These roles are:

1. Watchdog to monitor informed consent situations
2. Advocate to mediate on behalf of patients
3. Resource person to provide information on alternatives
4. Coordinator to preserve an open, friendly atmosphere for discussion
5. Facilitator to clarify differences between involved parties

Such studies raise the larger issue of disclosure of information in informed consent. Questions arise about what information should be disclosed, how much, and by whom. One study on the attitudes of nurses and medical students toward nurses disclosing information to patients pointed to areas of possible conflict. Generally, this conflict can be seen as one between a strong view of patients' rights and the need of hospital structures to maintain singular, orderly channels of communication (Davis & Jameton, 1987).

The nurse's ethical obligation in informed consent is to ascertain whether the patient understands what he or she has been told and what has been consented to. Informed consent is an imperfect tool and patients may have questions about the research or treatment they have agreed to. Even if the patients do not initiate this subject, the nurse needs to assess whether patients actually do understand the nature of the treatment regimen.

Informed consent applies as much to nursing interventions as it does to those of medicine. While implied consent may be inferred simply by the patient's presence in the care delivery setting, nurses must not neglect to obtain express consent wherever possible. That is, nurses should remain in a fluid relationship of full informedness and freely expressed consent for nursing care to the greatest extent possible.

Once the nurse has discovered that the patient does not understand aspects of the treatment, the nurse's ethical obligation is to report this to the physician so that he or she can meet the ethical obligation to inform. Usually, physicians follow through and speak further with patients regarding their treatment. If a physician decides not to provide additional information, however, or not to clarify what has already been said, the question arises as to the nurse's obligation in the situation. Has the nurse met the professional obligation by telling the physician that the patient needs additional input about treatment, or does he or she need to do something more when the physician does not follow through? Yes, something more needs to be done. The nurse's primary commitment is to the patient, as the ANA *Code of Ethics* declares. The *Code* further states:

> Patients have a moral and legal right to determine what will be done with their own person; to be given accurate, complete, and understandable information in a manner that facilitates an informed judgment; to be assisted with weighing the benefits, burdens, and available options in their treatment, including the choice of no treatment; to accept, refuse, or terminate treatment without deceit, undue influence, duress, coercion, or penalty; and to be given necessary support throughout the decision-making and treatment process. (ANA, 2001, pp. 8–10)

CASE STUDY I.

Marjorie is a spry and independent woman. She is very strong minded and practical. At the age of 87, she is diagnosed with pancreatic cancer, and a Whipple operation is offered as a potential cure. Her surgeon carefully explains to her the risks of the procedure, which, given her age, include the real possibility of death. As she understands the situation, she will either die a lingering death from cancer, she will be cured by the surgery, or she will die "under the knife." She consents to the surgery. She gets her affairs in order and appoints a conservator to manage her financial affairs.

Marjorie does not die on the table but she lingers for seven months in the intensive care unit as a result of successive complications. She is conscious, but unable to communicate. As is typical in these complex medical situations, each physiological problem is addressed individually. Therefore, each of Marjorie's complications was considered "potentially treatable," since her cancer was gone.

The nurses were disturbed by Marjorie's prolonged suffering, as were her friends. They questioned if she really understood the potential consequences of such a radical surgery. Their concerns were discussed with her physicians, who justified the continued aggressive treatment on the grounds that she must want this since she had agreed to such radical treatment in the first place.

Suggested Questions for Discussion

1. How do you understand what the patient is consenting to and what difference does this make?
2. Was her consent informed?
3. Do physicians and nurses understand informed consent differently? If so, why?

CASE STUDY II.

Ms Y is a 34-year-old woman who has been under medical care for a severe seizure disorder. During one of her medical visits, her physician discusses advance directives with her. He advises her to complete one because her seizures are likely to worsen and leave her incapacitated in the future. She does so and appoints her mother, Mrs. X, who has a fifth-grade education, as her designee on her durable power of attorney for health care form.

One month later, Ms Y has a devastating seizure. Her mother is present in the emergency room, where the physicians repeatedly seek her consent to provide emergency care, including placing Ms Y on a ventilator and other forms of life support. Mrs. X asks if the ventilator is life support, saying, "That ain't life support is it? She doesn't want life support." She is told it is not life support and that it is used to make Ms Y comfortable. Ms Y stays in a coma for two months, from which she emerges totally incapacitated; she must be fed, bathed, and diapered. She can speak only a few words such as "water" and "bury me," must be tied to the bed because she thrashes around violently, and screams for many hours each day.

Suggested Questions for Discussion

1. When is consent informed?
2. What are the assumptions we make regarding the average person's understanding of the practice of medicine and how hospitals work? How does this affect the process of informed consent?
3. What other factors influence the process of informed consent? Do you think Mrs. X's educational level was a factor here?
4. Should health care providers even attempt to engage in the process of informed consent in emergency situations?

Notes

1. *Fortner v Koch.* 272 Mich 273, 282, 261, NW (Mich 1935).
2. *Grants Administration Manual.* United States Department of Health, Education and Welfare, 1971.
3. The World Medical Association. *Declaration of Helsinki on Ethical Principles for Medical Research Involving Human Subjects, as adopted by the 52nd WMA General Assembly,* Edinburgh, October 2008.

References

Abdellah, F. G. (1967). Approaches to protecting the rights of human subjects. *Nursing Research, 16*(4), 316–320.

Alderson, P. (1995). Consent and the social context. *Nursing Ethics, 2*(4), 347–350.

Alt-White, A. (1995). Obtaining "informed" consent from the elderly. *Western Journal of Nursing Research, 17*(6), 700–705.

American Nurses Association Committee on Research and Studies. (1968). The nurse in research: ANA guidelines on ethical values. *Nursing Research, 17,* 104–107.

American Nurses Association. (2001). *Code of ethics for nurses with interpretive statements* (pp. 12–13). Silver Spring, MD: American Nurses Association, Provision 3.3.

American Nurses Association Commission on Nursing Research (1975): *Human Rights Guidelines for Nurses in Clinical and Other Research.* Kansas City, MO: American Nurses Association.

Appelbaum, P. S., & Grisso, T. (1988). Assessing patients' capacities to consent to treatment. *New England Journal of Medicine, 319,* 1635–1638.

Aveyard, H. (2005, January). Informed consent prior to nursing care procedures. *Nursing Ethics, 12*(1), 19–29.

Barber, B. (1976). The ethics of experimentation with human subjects. *Scientific American, 234,* 25–31.

Barrett, R. (2005, July). Quality of informed consent: measuring understanding among participants in oncology clinical trials. *Oncology Nursing Forum, 32*(4), 751–755.

Batey, M. V. (1970). Some methodological issues in research. *Nursing Research, 19,* 511–516.

Baumrind, D. (1973). Principles of ethical conduct in the treatment of subjects. *American Psychologist, 27,* 1083.

Beauchamp, T., & Childress, J. (2001). *Principles of biomedical ethics* (5th ed., pp. 176–188). New York: Oxford University Press.

Beecher, H. (1966). Ethics and clinical research. *New England Journal of Medicine, 274*(24), 1354–1360.

Bernard, C. (1927). *An introduction to the study of experimental medicine.* New York: Macmillan.

Berthold, J. S. (1969). Advancement of science and technology while maintaining human rights and values. *Nursing Research, 18,* 514–522.

Blackhall, L. J., Murphy, S. T., Frank, G., Michel, V., & Azen, S. (1995). Ethnicity and attitudes toward patient autonomy. *JAMA, 274*(10), 820–825.

Brody, H. (1992). *The healer's power.* New Haven, CT: Yale University Press.

Brody, H. (1995). The best system in the world. *Hastings Center Report, 25*(6 Suppl.), S18–S21.

Broome, M., & Stieglitz, K. (1992). The consent process and children. *Research in Nursing and Health, 15*(2), 147–152.

Butterworth, C. (2005, January 26–February 1). Ongoing consent to care for older people in care homes. *Nursing Standard, 19*(20), 40–45.

Callahan, D. (1994). Bioethics: Private choice and common good. *Hastings Center Report, 24*(3), 28–31.

Cantini, F., & Ells, C. (2007, June). The role of the clinical trial nurse in the informed consent process. *Canadian Jour of Nursing Research, 39*(2), 126–144.

Caplan, A. L. (1989). In brief—The meaning of the Holocaust for bioethics. *Hastings Center Report, 19*(4), 2–3.

Carrese, J. A., & Rhodes, L. A. (1995). Western bioethics on the Navajo reservation: Benefit or harm? *JAMA, 274*(10), 826–829.

Cohn, E., & Larsen, E. (2007, 3rd qtr). Improving participant comprehension in the informed consent process. *Journal of Nursing Scholarship, 39*(3), 273–280.

Community Practitioner. (2005, March). Consent for screening and immunisation procedures in children and young people. *Community Practitioner, 78*(3), 83–84.

Council on Ethical and Judicial Affairs. (1995). American Medical Association: Ethical issues in managed care. *JAMA, 273*(4), 330–335.

Crowley, M., & Connors, D. (1985). Critique of "The use of animals in research." *Advances in Nursing Science, 7*(4), 23–31.

Cunningham, S., & Mitchell, P. (1982). The use of animals in nursing research. *Advances in Nursing Science, 4*(4), 72–84.

Curtin, L. (1993). Informed consent: Cautious, calculated candor. *Nursing Management, 24*(4), 18–20.

Davis, A. J. (1988). The clinical nurse's role in informed consent. *Journal of Professional Nursing, 4,* 88–91.

Davis, A. J. (1989a). Informed consent process in research protocols: Dilemmas for clinical nurses. *Western Journal of Nursing Research, 11,* 448–457.

Davis, A. J. (1989b). Clinical nurses ethical decision making in situations of informed consent. *ANS. Advances in Nursing Science, 11*(3), 63–69.

Davis, A. (1992, August 22). *Nursing's role in creating the ideal society.* Presented at the conference, The Value of the Human Being: Medicine Under the Nazis, San Francisco, CA.

Davis, A. J., & Koenig, B. A. (1996). A question of policy: Bioethics in a multicultural society. *Nursing Policy Forum, 2*(1), 6–11.

Davis, A. J., & Krueger, J. C. (1980). *Patients, nurses, ethics.* New York: American Journal of Nursing Company.

Davis, A. J., & Jameton, A. (1987). Nursing and medical student attitudes toward nursing disclosure of information to patients: A pilot study. *Journal of Advanced Nursing, 12*(6), 691–698.

Donovan, J. (1990). Animal rights and feminist theory. *Signs, 15*(2), 350–375.

Donnelley, S. (1995). Bioethical troubles: Animal individuals and human organisms. *Hastings Center Report, 25*(7), 21–29.

Ehrenreich, B., & Ehrenreich, J. (1990). The system behind the chaos. In N. McKenzie (Ed.), *The crisis in health care: Ethical issues* (pp. 50–69). New York: Meridian.

Erlen, J. (1994a). Informed consent: The information component. *Orthopaedic Nursing, 13*(2), 75–78.

Erlen, J. (1994b). Informed consent: The consent component. *Orthopaedic Nursing, 13*(4), 65–67.

Erlen, J. (1995). When the patient lacks decision-making capacity. *Orthopaedic Nursing, 14*(4), 51–54.

Faden, R. R., & Beauchamp, J. (1986). *A history and theory of informed consent.* New York: Oxford University press.

Fowler, M. (1988). Pediatric informed consent. *Heart Lung, 17,* 584–585.

Fox, R., & Swazey, J. (1992). Leaving the field. *Hastings Center Report, 22*(5), 9–15.

Grace, P. J., McLaughlin, M. (2005, April). Ethical issues. When consent isn't informed enough: what's the nurse's role when a patient has given consent but doesn't fully understand the risks? *American Journal of Nursing, 105*(4), 79, 81–84.

Gray, B. H. (1975). *Human subjects in medical experimentation.* New York: Wiley.

Grebe, R. (2007, December). Informed consent for patients with cognitive impairment. *Nurse Practitioner, 32*(12), 39–44.

Haggerty, L. A., & Hawkins, J. (2000, June). Informed consent and the limits of confidentiality. *Western Journal of Nursing Research, 22*(4), 508–514.

Hayes, M. O. (2006, Summer). Prisoners and autonomy: implications for the informed consent process with vulnerable populations. *Journal of Forensic Nursing, 2*(2), 84–89.

Hofling, C., Brotzman, E., Dalrymple, S., et al. (1966). An experimental study in nursepatient relationships. *Journal of Nervous and Mental Disease, 143,* 171–180.

Holloway, I., & Wheeler, S. (1995). Ethical issues in qualitative health research. *Nursing Ethics, 2*(3), 223–232.

Holmes, H., & Purdy, L. (1992). *Feminist perspectives in medical ethics.* Bloomington, IN: Indiana University Press.

Humphreys, L. (1970). *Tearoom trade: Impersonal sex in public places.* Chicago: Aldine.

Imbus, S., & Zawacki, B. (1977). Autonomy for burned patients when survival is unprecedented. *New England Journal of Medicine, 297*(6), 308–311.

Jonas, H. (1969). Philosophical reflections on experimenting with human subjects. In P. A. Freund (Ed.), *Experimentation with human subjects* (pp. 1–31). New York: Braziller.

Kant, I. (1964). *Groundwork of the metaphysics of morals.* New York: Harper Torchbooks.

Katz, J. (1993). Ethics in clinical research revisited. *Hastings Center Report, 23*(5), 31–39.

Koenig, B. A., & Marshall, P. (1994, December 2). *Bioethics and the politics of race and ethnicity: Respecting (or constructing) Difference?* Paper presented at "Cultural Diversity and Bioethics," American Anthropological Association Annual Meeting, Atlanta, GA.

Kuz, K. M. (2006, June) Young teenagers providing their own surgical consents: an ethical-legal dilemma for perioperative registered nurses. *Canadian Operating Room Nursing Journal, 24*(2), 6–8, 10–1, 14–5.

Liaschenko, J. (1994). The moral geography of home care. *Advances in Nursing Science, 17*(2), 16–26.

Liaschenko, J. (1995). Artificial personhood: Nursing ethics in a medical world. *Nursing Ethics, 2*(3), 185–196.

Lifton, R. J. (1986). *The Nazi Doctors: Medical killing and the psychology of genocide.* New York: Basic Books.

Lorenzen, B., Melby, C., & Earles, B. (2008, July). Using principles of health literacy to enhance the informed consent process. *AORN Journal, 88*(1), 23–29.

Markowitz, M. S. (1993). Human fetal tissue: Ethical implications for use in research and therapy. *AWHONNS Clinical Issues in Perinatal and Womens Health Nursing, 4*(4), 578–588.

Mathar, H., & Morville, A. (2006, October). Autonomy and Informed consent in Nursing. *Klinisk Sygepleje, 20*(4), 59–66.

McGrath, P. (1995). It's ok to say no! A discussion of ethical issues arising from informed consent to chemotherapy. *Cancer Nursing, 18*(2), 97–103.

McKenzie, N. (Ed.). (1990). The new ethical demand in the crisis of primary care medicine. *The crisis in health care: Ethical issues* (pp. 113–126). New York: Meridian.

McMullen, P., & Philipsen, N. (1993). Informed consent: It's more than just a signature on paper. *Nursing Connections, 9*(2), 41–43.

Menzel, P. (1990). *Strong medicine: The ethical rationing of health care.* New York: Oxford University Press.

Miller, B. (1981). Autonomy and the refusal of lifesaving treatment. *Hastings Center Report, 11*(4), 22–28.

Morreim, E. H. (1995a). *Balancing acts: The new medical ethics of medicine's new economics.* Washington, DC: Georgetown University Press.

Morreim, E. H. (1995b). The ethics of incentives in managed care. *Trends Health Care Law Ethics, 10*(1–2), 57–62.

Nelson, J. L. (1992). Transplantation through a glass darkly. *Hastings Center Report, 22*(5), 6–8.

Nokes, K. M., & Nwakeze, P. C. (2007, November). Assessing cognitive capacity for participation in a research study. *Clinical Nursing Research, 16*(4), 336–349.

Orona, C. J., Koenig, B. A., & Davis, A. J. (1994). Cultural issues in nondisclosure. *Cambridge Quarterly of Healthcare Ethics, 3*(3), 338–346.

Proctor, R. (1988). *Racial hygiene: Medicine under the Nazis.* Cambridge, MA: Harvard University Press.

Parsons, T. (1951). *The social system.* Glencoe, IL: Free Press.

Pérez, J. L., & Borbolla, F. J. R. (2007, May). Basis for the elaboration of an informed consent form in nursing. *Metas de Enfermeria, 10*(4), 63–70.

Presidents Commission for the Study of Ethical Problems in Medicine and Biomedical and Behavioral Research (2005): *Making Health Care Decisions.* Washington, DC: United States Government Printing Office, 1982.

Reiser, S. J. (1994). The ethical life of health care organizations. *Hastings Center Report, 24*(6), 28–35.

Roberson, A. J. (2007). Adolescent informed consent: ethics, law, and theory to guide policy and nursing research. *Journal of Nursing Law, 11*(4), 191–196.

Rodwin, M. A. (1993). *Medicine, money, and morals: Physicians' conflicts of interest.* New York: Oxford University Press.

Rodwin, M. A. (1995). Conflicts in managed care. *New England Journal of Medicine, 332*(9), 604–607.

Rosenhan, D. L. (1973). On being sane in insane places. *Science, 167*, 250–258.

Sanders, L. M., Giudice, L., & Raffin. T. (1993). Ethics of fetal tissue transplantation. *Western Journal of Medicine, 159*(3), 400–407.

Schwartz, S. I. (1979). Consensus summary on fluid resuscitation. *Journal of Trauma, 19*(suppl), 876–877.

Shaibu, S. (2007, July). Ethical and cultural considerations in informed consent in Botswana. *Nursing Ethics, 14*(4), 503–509.

Silva, M. C. (1993). Competency, comprehension, and the ethics of informed consent. *Nursing Connections, 6*(3), 47–51.

Silva, M. C. (1995a). *Ethical guidelines in the conduct, dissemination, and implementation of nursing research.* Washington, DC: American Nurses Association Publishing.

Silva, M. C. (1995b). *Annotated bibliography for ethical guidelines.* Washington, DC: American Nurses Association Publishing.

Seidelman, W. (1989). In memoriam: Medicine's confrontation with evil. *Hastings Center Report, 19*(6), 5–6.

Slaughter, S., Cole, D., Jennings, E., Reamer, M. A. (2007, January). Consent and assent to participate in research from people with dementia. *Nursing Ethics, 14*(1), 27–40.

Sherwin, S. (1992). *No longer patient: Feminist ethics and health care.* Philadelphia: Temple University Press.

Shorr, A. S. (1994). Abortion and fetal research: Some ethical concerns. *Fetal Diagnosis and Therapy, 9*(3), 196–203.

Spitz, V. (2005). *Doctors from Hell: The horrific account of Nazi experiments on humans.* Boulder, CO: Sentient Press.

Steppe, H. (1991). Nursing in the Third Reich. *History of Nursing Society Journal, 3*(4), 21–37.

Steppe, H. (1992). Nursing in Nazi Germany. *Western Journal of Nursing Research, 14*(6), 744–753.

Tabak, N., & Zvi, M. R. (2008, March–May). When parents refuse a sick teenager the right to give informed consent: the nurse's role. *Australian Journal of Advanced Nursing, 25*(3), 106–111.

Teasdale, K., & Kent, G. (1995). The use of deception in nursing. *Journal of Medical Ethics, 21* (2), 77–81.

Thurber, F., Deatrick, J., & Grey, M. (1992). children's participation in research: Their right to consent. *Journal of Pediatric Nursing, 7*(3), 165–170.

Tillett, J. (2005, April–June). Adolescents and informed consent: Ethical and legal issues. *Journal of Perinatal and Neonatal Nursing, 19*(2), 112–121.

Trials of War Criminals before the Nuremberg Military Tribunals under Control Council Law (1949) No. 10, Vol. 2, pp. 181–182. Washington, DC: U.S. Government Printing Office.

Wear, S. (1993). *Informed consent: Patient autonomy and physician benefience within clinical medicine.* Dordrecht: Kluwer Academic Publishers.

Winslow, B., & Winslow, G. (1991). Integrity and compromise in nursing ethics. *The Journal of medicine and philosophy, 16,* 307–323.

White, B. C. (1994). *Competence to consent.* Washington, DC: Georgetown University Press.

Yamokoski, A. D., Hazen, R. A., & Kodish, E. D. (2008, January–February). Anticipatory guidance to improve informed consent: a new application of the concept. *Journal of Pediatric Oncology Nursing, 25*(1), 34–43.

CHAPTER 7

Abortion

INTRODUCTION

The field of reproductive technology has exploded in recent years. Neonatal intensive care is a dramatic example of high-technology medicine and nursing. Embryo freezing as an adjunct to in vitro fertilization (IVF) is another technique in the treatment of infertility and control of human reproduction. Technologies such as artificial insemination, IVF, surrogate motherhood, and ovum transfer raise numerous ethical issues. Among these developments fetal research and surgery have received much attention as an ethical concern in public policy. Experimental drugs and other chemicals used to terminate early pregnancy raise the question about the status of the early embryo. And yet, with all these scientific developments and the attending ethical dilemmas raised by them, it is the ancient act of abortion that holds center stage in the debates over the control of reproduction.

Abortion, the expulsion or removal of the embryo from the uterus, generally occurs before the 28th week of pregnancy. Spontaneous abortion occurs as a result of a variety of endogenous and exogenous causes, excluding intentional human action. Induced abortion to deliberately terminate a pregnancy, performed either legally or illegally, relies on numerous different methods. The method used depends, in part, on timing, or how long the woman has been pregnant. Medically speaking, abortion during the first trimester is the easiest to perform and the safest for the woman involved. However, women do undergo abortion during the second trimester and even up to fetus viability, which means that it has the potential ability to live outside the uterus, albeit with artificial means, if necessary. Traditionally, viability was thought to occur around 28 weeks, but technological developments have moved the time to an earlier date in the pregnancy. In the last trimester, abortion presents increased dangers to the woman, and the likelihood of delivering a viable fetus also increases. However, abortion during the third trimester is sometimes considered in cases of severe fetal abnormality or life-threatening risk to the woman.

Abortion, an ancient form of birth control, has been used worldwide for centuries. Now it can be argued that other effective contraceptive methods have been developed that could replace abortion as a means of birth control in many cases. These alternatives to abortion have the potential of presenting fewer ethical dilemmas. However, several factors must be taken into account before pursuing this line of argument very far. First, not all people receive sound knowledge about sex and reproduction, and in some places, people still continue the debate over sex education in schools. Second, some questions have been raised regarding the safety of the most effective birth control device, the contraceptive pill, for some women. And finally, the fact remains that people do not necessarily act on the information and knowledge they have, even when the results of their actions may prove detrimental to their health or lives. Behaviors such as smoking, driving while intoxicated, indulging in unprotected sex in the era of AIDS, and having sexual intercourse without using some form of contraception when the couple does not want a pregnancy all support this observation. Contraceptive devices succeed in preventing unwanted pregnancies only if used consistently. The nature of human sexuality and the complex motivations that people bring to their sexual experiences favor mishaps. So for these and myriad other reasons, abortion as a form of birth control remains with us.

Few other recent topics have caused so much outcry and agitation, although assisted suicide may do so in the future. One side of the debate has been called *the right to life* or *pro-life,* while the other side is known as *the right to choice* or *pro-choice.* Many people take a position somewhere between these two stances but are not so visible or vocal in their ethical position. The ethical dilemmas in abortion are complex and require a careful examination. It seems reasonable to assume that this examination will take into account the social and religious diversity in the United States and will recall that a major legal basis is the separation of church and state. Many factors intersect in any discussion of abortion: medical, sociological, psychological, technological, legal, and the attitudes and values grounded in philosophical and moral concerns of the public. This background information, along with an overview of the historical and social context of abortion, will help us to understand more fully the ethical dilemmas surrounding abortion.

THE RELIGIOUS AND HISTORICAL CONTEXT

During the Persian Empire, abortifacients were accessible, though individuals who performed criminal abortions received severe punishment. In ancient Greece and during the Roman era, people resorted to abortion without scruple in part because of the belief that the fetus was not immediately ensouled with a human soul. Plato in *The Republic* and Aristotle in *Politics* described abortion as a means of preventing excess population. Neither Greek nor Roman law afforded protection to the unborn fetus. Furthermore, the religions practiced in these cultures did not ban abortion (or infanticide by exposure); however, philosophers, religious teachers, and physicians debated the morality of performing abortions. In this climate, the Hippocratic Oath developed and took a position against abortion. This radical departure from the prevailing practice may have been influenced by Pythagorean dogma. Most Greek thinkers, except for the Pythagorean School, commended abortion, at least prior to viability. For the Pythagoreans, the embryo became animated or infused with a soul from the moment of conception, so that abortion meant destroying a living being. The abortion clause in the Hippocratic Oath reflects Pythagorean doctrine, a small segment of Greek opinion at the time. However, medical writings down to Galen's time (AD 130–200) provided evidence of violation of almost every injunction of the oath. Only at the end of antiquity, with the emerging teachings of Christianity, which agreed with the Pythagorean ethic, did the oath become the nucleus of all medical ethics.

The Greco-Roman world, distinguished by its indifference to fetal life, also saw the development of Christianity give rise to values in opposition to and in conflict with the generally held popular beliefs. Early Christian teachings on sexuality and abortion developed in part as a means of resistance to the oppression and political influence of the Roman Empire. To adopt different attitudes toward sexuality and abortion was to repudiate Roman power. The specific Christian teaching on abortion was grounded in the Old Testament command to love your neighbor as yourself (Leviticus 19:18). The basis for fulfillment of this commandment, found in the New Testament, emphasized the sacrifice of a one's life for another (John 15:13). From this commandment of love, the Christian valuation of human life evolved.

Abortion, as a subject of concern to secular humanists and theologians, has a long history. At the heart of this complex discourse lies the question of how one determines the humanity of a being. The Roman Catholic position on abortion has been clearly stated since the late 1880s and has been reaffirmed by recent popes. Roman Catholics, and other religious leaders, believe that the embryo becomes a human being with a soul from the moment of fertilization. Some of the early teachers of the Church, however, including St. Thomas Aquinas, did not consider an unformed embryo to have a soul and placed ensoulment at about 3 months after conception, when the fetus had developed a recognizable human shape. Along with this concept of ensoulment at conception, Roman Catholics reject abortion on the grounds that unborn children need baptism. Although not as strongly asserted in the Church today, this doctrine of baptizing the endangered fetus still holds. The current official position of Catholic leaders accepts the concept of ensoulment that defines the fetus as a human being from fertilization. This position is a refusal to discriminate among human beings on the basis of their varying potentialities.

Protestant views vary according to the numerous denominations and groups involved. Although many Protestants do not agree with the Roman Catholic Church on ensoulment, they do regard abortion as undesirable, since the embryo as an entity should be preserved from unnecessary destruction. Generally, for Protestants, the concept of the sacredness of life has served as an obstacle to the wanton, thoughtless, or convenience performance of abortion. In attempting to determine when human life begins, most Protestant leaders agree that by the time of quickening, or the first recognizable movements of the fetus in utero, one can define the fetus as a human being, though this does not specifically resolve the question about abortion.

Pertinent principles can be stipulated for reflection and reduced to the following simplified scheme. First, life ought to be preserved rather than destroyed; second, protection must be provided, especially to those who cannot assert their own right to life; and third, exceptions to these rules exist, such as (a) medical indications that make therapeutic abortion morally tolerable, (b) pregnancy resulting from a sexual assault or incest, and (c) social and emotional conditions that do not appear beneficial for the well-being of the mother and child. This scheme replaces the determination of an action as right or wrong according to its conformity to a rule and its application with stressing the primacy of the person and human relationships along with the concreteness of the choice within limited possibilities. In the case of abortion, no guarantee of an objectively right action can be given, since several values, all objectively important, exist. These values do not resolve themselves into a harmonious relationship with each other. Since there is no single overriding determination of what constitutes a right action, there can be no unambiguously right act.

Ancient Jewish writings consider the fetus a living being when it detaches itself from the mother. According to the Talmud, this occurs when the head has emerged from the birth canal. In more modern times, Orthodox Jewish leaders maintain that abortion is morally wrong at any time, except when the mother's life becomes seriously threatened. Reform Jews accept more reasons for abortion. For all practical purposes, the relatively permissive attitudes of Conservative and Reform Judaism can be equated with those of a growing number of Protestant denominations on the topic of abortion. Buddhists condemn killing of the fetus but define commencement of life rather loosely, whereas the Shinto religion recognizes the infant as a living being only after its birth. The Islamic religion takes the stance that abortion is permissible until the embryo develops into the human shape at 120 days after conception (Riddle, 1994, 1997).

THE LEGAL AND POLITICAL CONTEXT

The legal aspects of abortion have been influenced by religious developments and definitions. In the fourth century AD, the Roman Empire developed the first laws against abortion in a time when Christian influence began to be felt. However, in common law, abortion performed before quickening, at 16–18 weeks, was not an indictable offense. This lack of criminality in common law for abortion occurring before quickening was influenced by theological concepts, civil and canonical law concepts, and philosophical concepts of the beginning of life—or when the embryo becomes infused with a soul. Christian theology and canon law fixed the point of animation at 40 days for a male and 80 days for a female, a view that persisted until the 19th century. General agreement developed that prior to animation, the fetus was part of the mother and therefore its destruction was not homicide. However, because of the uncertainty as to the exact time of animation, and perhaps influenced by Aquinas' definition of movement in utero as one criterion of life, Bracton wrote in 1640 in the first references to abortion in English criminal law that to abort a woman is homicide if the embryo is formed and especially if it is animated. Other English legal scholars used the concept of quickening to develop the common law precedents regarding abortion. In 1803, England's first criminal abortion statute made the abortion of a quick fetus a capital crime. This law also provided lesser penalties for the felony of abortion that occurred before quickening. In 1967, the British Parliament enacted a new, liberal abortion law (Landis, 2006).

In the United States, generally speaking, the law in effect until the middle of the 19th century was the preexisting English common law. In 1800, abortions were not prohibited in American jurisdictions, but this progressively changed over the next century with the first antiabortion laws being introduced between 1821 and 1841. During the middle and late 19th century, the distinction based on quickening disappeared from the statutory law in most states, and the penalties for performing an abortion increased. For approximately 100 years, the United States outlawed virtually all abortions, but demand for abortion as well as the untoward consequences of illegal abortions changed this policy so that by the early 1970s only the states of Louisiana, New Hampshire, and Pennsylvania prohibited abortion for any reason. This is in contrast to the following state laws: Alaska, Hawaii, New York, Washington, and the District of Columbia permitted it for any reason; 13 states allowed abortion to protect the physical and mental health of the mother; one state permitted abortion only on the grounds of saving the woman's life and in cases of rape; and 29 states sanctioned it only to save the woman's life. Colorado pioneered this liberalizing trend in abortion laws in 1967, and rather than creating an abortion-mill situation, as feared by its critics, this statute resulted in caution on the part of physicians and hospitals (Landis, 2006).

Texas was the residence of Jane Roe, a pseudonym for Norma McCorvey, and became the proving ground for abortion rights in this country. Roe could not obtain an abortion because her pregnancy was not life threatening, a criterion for abortion in Texas. She sued the state of Texas, filing a class action suit. The U.S. Supreme Court decision, delivered on January 22, 1973, declared both an original statute (Texas, *Roe v Wade*) and a reform statute (Georgia, *Doe v Bolton*) unconstitutional. The decision by the majority of seven to two of the Supreme Court justices asserted that the constitutional right to privacy, provided for by the Fourteenth Amendment, is broad enough to encompass a woman's decision whether or not to terminate her pregnancy. Furthermore, a state cannot interfere in the abortion decision between a woman and her physician during the first trimester. In the second trimester, when abortion becomes more hazardous, the state's interest in the woman's health permits the enactment of regulation to protect maternal health. Beyond these procedural requirements, the abortion decision still rests with the woman and her physician. After the fetus reaches viability, approximately in the last trimester, the state can exercise its interest in promoting potential human life. Then, the state can prohibit abortion except when the necessity arises to preserve the life or health of the mother. The Court did not support the position that a woman has an absolute right to abortion regardless of circumstances; however, the position it took did make legal abortion potentially more available than at any time in the United States during the 20th century.[1]

According to the Guttmacher Institute July 2008 statistics, almost half of pregnancies among American women are unintended, and 4 in 10 of these are terminated by abortion; 22 percent of all pregnancies end in abortions. In 2005, 1.21 million abortions were performed down from 1.31 million in 2000. Fifty percent of women obtaining abortions are younger than 25.[2]

We have, for obvious reasons, fewer facts about illegal abortions that occurred prior to the 1973 legal change. However, some observations have been made that suggest certain patterns and concerns. In the United States before the 1973 Supreme Court decision, abortion was largely performed clandestinely by physicians, especially for the financially well-off. The poor were more likely to abort themselves or to resort to nonmedical amateurs. As well as can be determined, the majority of those fetuses aborted were from married women with several children. Death and invalidism have not been insignificant as an aftermath of illegal abortion. In the 1960s, almost 50 percent of deaths in New York City associated with pregnancy and childbirth resulted from illegal abortions (Legge, 1985).

Pro-choice persons continue to fight to remove the remaining restrictions in abortion law, while antiabortionists strive for a constitutional amendment that would recognize that a fetus has rights, including a right to life. Efforts to overturn the 1973 *Roe v Wade* decision by constitutional amendments have failed to date, but another strategy, the passage of state abortion statutes that are as restrictive as possible within the *Roe v Wade* framework, aim to see the Supreme Court ultimately modify or abandon *Roe* altogether. Such challenges have gone to the Supreme Court nearly every year. For the Court to permit states to outlaw abortion—the most frequently performed medical procedure in the United States—seems unlikely, but a narrowing of *Roe* seems possible. Other strategies have included congressional measures to limit abortions. For example, in the late 1970s, Congress prohibited the use of Medicaid funds for abortions, except when the woman's life is endangered, thus limiting access for poor women. More recent attempts to limit *Roe v Wade* concern restrictions to minors seeking abortions and attempts to confine abortions to earlier points in pregnancy. In light of its long history and the great passions generated by the issue of abortion, continuation of this controversy can be expected in and out of legislatures and courts (Landis, 2006).

The battle over abortion, called the battle of life versus choice, has become one of the most emotional issues of politics and morality facing the United States today. The language used in this debate is so passionate and polemical, and the conflicting and seemingly irreconcilable values so deeply felt, that this issue could well test the very foundations of a pluralistic system of government that was designed to accommodate deep-rooted moral and ethical differences. This was made dramatically clear with the murders of physicians and staff at family planning clinics in different parts of the country a few years ago. It is possible that nothing since the issue of slavery has the potential of dividing us in our quest for a democratic society as much as abortion.

Some believe that abortion is murder of an unborn person and therefore should be outlawed by constitutional amendment. Others argue that abortion is a legal right that women must have because they must be free to control their bodies and their lives. Along with the ethical dilemma of abortion itself, another issue, that of the government's role, has become paramount. Should abortion be legal or illegal? If legal, should government funds be available to cover the cost of abortion for the poor? The issue of abortion continues to be a major political battle of the early 21st century.

THE MEDICAL AND SCIENTIFIC CONTEXT

Institutionalized medicine has tremendous influence on the control of reproduction in general and abortion in particular. It is not surprising to learn that historically medicine as a profession has been extremely conservative in its sociopolitical views. The medical profession shared the antiabortion mood prevalent in the United States during the latter part of the 19th century and may have influenced the enactment of stringent criminal abortion legislation. In 1857, the American Medical Association (AMA) appointed a Committee on Criminal Abortion to investigate criminal abortion with a view to its general suppression. In 1859, this committee proposed, and the AMA adopted, a resolution against unwarrantable destruction of human life. They called upon state legislatures to revise their abortion laws and requested the cooperation of state medical societies in pressing the subject. The committee, in 1871, again proposed resolutions that the AMA adopted. This time one recommendation read that it "be unlawful and unprofessional for any physician to induce abortion or premature labor without the concurrent opinion of at least one respectable consulting physician, and then always with a view to the safety of the child—if that be possible." They also recommended calling "the attention of the clergy of all denominations to the perverted views of morality entertained by a large class of females—aye, and men also, on this important question."[3]

Except for occasional condemnation of criminal abortionists, the AMA took no further formal action on abortion until 1967, when the Committee on Human Reproduction urged adoption of a policy in which the Association would oppose induced abortion except where (a) documented medical evidence showed a threat to the health or life of the mother, (b) the child may be born with incapacitating physical deformity or mental disorder, or (c) a pregnancy resulting from legally established statutory or forcible rape or incest may constitute a threat to the physical or mental health of the patient. In addition, the committee proposed that two other physicians with recognized professional competency examine the patient and concur in writing to the need for the abortion and that the physician perform the abortion in a hospital accredited by the Joint Commission on Accreditation of Hospitals. The AMA House of Delegates adopted this policy. In 1970, the resolutions before the House of Delegates did not differ from the policy adopted in 1967 with the exception of the statement that "no party to the procedure should be requested to violate personally held moral principles" (American Medical Association, 1967, 1970).

The reason for the change in the medical profession's stance is unclear. One possible explanation is the increasing development of scientific knowledge as a basis for medicine in the 20th century. Traditional notions of ensoulment and personhood are seen as lying outside the province of science. Questions of viability do fall within the domain of scientific knowledge; however, this too can prove problematic.

Science, like religion, finds it difficult to establish the moment when life begins. One embryologist could define the unfertilized egg as a living entity, while another embryologist could indicate great limitations in that definition because the unfertilized egg cannot continue to live more than a few days, has only half the chromosome supply that other cells in the body have, and therefore, cannot develop without the addition of the sperm. This situation changes when an egg becomes fertilized by a sperm, and this change results in a complete chromosome complement. The process of division begins, and growth occurs rapidly; however, up to the sixth week of the embryo's existence, only an expert embryologist can tell whether the embryo is human or not. At the seventh week, human characteristics begin appearing, and by the 15th or 16th week, the mother can feel the movements of the fetus (quickening).

All along the way of this remarkable process, the embryo has what some call the marvelous gift of life, but others would argue that this is true only in the same sense that an animal or plant has life. The question remains as to when during this process this entity develops human life. No clear biological definition has been developed as to the beginning of human life. A larger philosophical question is whether physical life and personhood are the same things. Is it possible to have physical life and not have personhood?

Since the 1973 abortion decision, advances in neonatal care have made 25 weeks the generally accepted time of viability. With this scientific change, the utility of the concept of viability for drawing legal and policy lines for abortion has been called into question. The development of neonatal medicine allows for the treatment of imperiled or premature newborns that would have died if they were born even only a few years ago. Some of these neonates scarcely bear a physical resemblance to a human baby. This technological capacity raises the question for the abortion debate of how we can ethically justify attempting to save imperiled 22–25-week-old neonates, while accepting the abortion of perfectly healthy fetuses of the same gestational age. The difference hangs on the notion of whether or not children are wanted. In one case, we speak of a cherished baby and in the other, a product of conception. Some of the public and health care professionals find these distinctions troubling (Francome, 2004; Schoen, 2005).

THE ETHICAL DILEMMA OF ABORTION

Since the 1973 Supreme Court decision, some believed that further ethical debate would only be academic in the most pejorative sense of that word. Others, however, believed that moral distinctions can be made within the framework of the reformed law and that these distinctions can assist the individual in developing or maintaining a moral position on abortion. The ethical dilemma involved can be limited to three of its dimensions for the purpose of this discussion: (a) the rights of the fetus, (b) the rights and obligations of the mother, and (c) the rights and obligations of society.

RIGHTS OF THE FETUS

In presenting *Roe v Wade* before the Supreme Court, the lawyer argued that the Constitution does not define "person" in so many words. Although the 14th Amendment contains three references to person, there can be no assurance that they have any prenatal application. The lawyer concluded that *under the law*, the unborn fetus is not a person. One important dimension of this ethical dilemma, however, asks for a definition of human life and some determination of when we can recognize its presence, so that we can then place a value on it and weigh it against other values. In the present state of biological ignorance on the matter and philosophical pluralism, the premise that the fetus is a person can be neither proved nor disproved to the satisfaction of all. Therefore, no one can assert superior moral sensitivity over opponents, and neither moral claim can rightfully eliminate the other from the social or political arena (Hull & Hoffer, 2001).

Those concerned with what they consider a helpless minority, unborn fetuses, judge the direct, intentional taking of innocent human life as unacceptable. Some of the arguments supporting the personhood of the fetus are as follows: We should impute full human dignity to the nonviable fetus because it will become viable. Genetics tells us that we are what we become in every cell and attribute. Genetic data therefore provide us with a scientific approximation to the religious belief of ensoulment from conception. Others contend that the zygote is not a *potential* person but an *actual* person in a nonfunctioning state. They maintain that fetal life is simply the first phase of the continuum of human life, and so any distinction is arbitrary.

If we grant that from conception a fetus possesses humanity, we must then accord it all human rights, including the most basic one, the right to life. To kill the fetus, which possesses humanity, is murder, except, arguably, in the cases of war, self-defense, and capital punishment. Some use moral reasoning to raise the larger question of whether the life of the fetus should receive the same protection as other lives. Basically, they ask the question: Is killing the fetus, by whatever means, and for whatever reasons, to be thought of as killing a human being? By drawing the line between abortions performed early in pregnancy and those done later, some people develop the moral position that early abortions do not violate the principle of protection of life.

One basic moral principle that has received much attention in recent years, that of informed consent, must be addressed in this dilemma. If one defines the fetus as possessing humanity at any point along the developmental continuum before birth, then the question that must be asked is this: Who speaks for this human, by the use of what criteria, and who guards his or her rights in this matter so vital to existence? One argument, especially for the severely deformed fetus, says that if the fetus could speak under these circumstances, he or she would consent to abortion. This argument can also be used to support abortions for the unwanted child without deformity. If the parent(s) does not want the child, what quality of life can the child expect to have? Will this child more likely become a victim of child abuse? The central question in this quality-of-life argument turns on the location of the line to be drawn. The extreme situation of this line of argumentation can be found in the phenomenon of wrongful life suits—suits brought on behalf of the severely disabled child for suffering and damages attendant to being born. The premise of these suits is that the disability was known before birth and the child's suffering would have been prevented by abortion (Hull & Hoffer, 2001).

RIGHTS AND OBLIGATIONS OF THE PREGNANT WOMAN

The moral principle of respect for autonomy leads to the position that a woman has the right to control over her own body and the right to determine whether or not to bear a child. The dilemma arises out of the fact that the situation involves the woman and the embryo/fetus. According to some, no one has an absolute, clear-cut right to control his or her fate where others share it. The Court took this consideration into account in its debate before changing the abortion law, when it made distinctions between what is allowed during the three trimesters as the embryo develops into a viable fetus.

The question has been raised as to whether anyone, before or after birth, child or adult, has the right to continued dependence upon the bodily processes of another against that person's will. Some argue that a woman, pregnant as a result of rape, incest, or in spite of every precaution, has no obligation to continue the pregnancy. In this case, abortion is equated with cessation of continued biological support, and not with unjust killing. An involuntarily pregnant woman can cease her support of life to the fetus without moral infringement of its right to life. Even those who support this argument under the circumstances specified might have difficulty using it in the situation of pregnancies entered into voluntarily. In this latter situation, the obligation of the pregnant woman to the fetus could be defined differently, and abortion might be considered a less responsible moral choice. Some take the position that pregnant women, no matter what the circumstances of conception, have obligations toward the life and well-being of the fetus that overshadow any discussion of the woman's rights. In some discussions in certain political arenas, the woman as a variable is not considered. The variables discussed are the father, the fetus, and society. So we have a moral argument, where the stakes are high, in which some people support abortion on demand based on respect for the woman's autonomy. At the same time, we have people who oppose abortion except (perhaps) to save the life of the mother, based on the sanctity of life principle and the personhood of the fetus. In the extreme of this view, the fetus's life takes priority over that of the woman. To think in a simple way about this ethical dilemma, on the one hand, the fetus is viewed as an object or a thing, while on the other, the woman is viewed as an object or a thing. The political novel *The Handmaid's Tale* takes this woman-as-object idea and stretches it to a chilling conclusion. In doing so, the darker interconnections between politics and sex are illuminated (Atwood, 1987).

Throughout world history, reproduction has been tied to the transmission of property. In fact, what we would now recognize as marriage in the Western world had its origins in the 11th century as a means to determine and assure inheritance. State control of reproduction has an equally long history and control of reproduction and therefore of sexuality has been imposed on women to these ends. Contemporary feminist thinkers ask if buried deeply beneath the abortion discussion one can find unresolved attitudes toward sex in this country that are left over from early Puritan days. Any ethical system, including contemporary ones, presupposes a cosmology or a social order. Feminist scholarship has shown that many of the current arguments surrounding abortion and reproductive issues have underlying assumptions about the place of women in the world (Sherwin, 1992). One can only wonder what role this politicization of reproduction plays in the conservative stance of some religious groups who are not only opposed to abortion but also to birth control. Prior to her appointment as a Supreme Court Justice, Ruth Bader Ginsburg presented an interesting argument criticizing the reasoning behind *Roe v Wade.* Rather than the right to privacy as the basis for the decision, she argued that an appeal to the equal protection clause of the Constitution would have been more appropriate. Men have a distinct advantage over women in social and political advancement due to the unique ability of women to be burdened by pregnancy. This line of argument would have made a clear stand for gender equity based upon the constitutional right to equal protection under the law (Ginsburg, 1994).

The major focus in much of the writing on abortion has been on what a third party, such as a physician, may or may not do when a woman requests an abortion. What the pregnant woman may do legally and morally was deduced from what third parties may do in the situation. Treating the matter of what the pregnant woman may do in such a fashion does not grant her the status of person that others insist on so firmly for the fetus. The pregnant woman and the fetus were considered as a unity until the development of technology enabled the conceptualization and ultimate visualization of the fetus as a separate entity. This has led some to view the woman as merely a fetal container. Witness the now famous cases in which brain-dead pregnant women (cadaveric pregnancies) have been maintained as physiological incubators until the living fetus could be delivered.

Traditionally, little attention has been given to the role, rights, and obligations of the father in the abortion decision. This reflects the law's concern with the individual, in this case the pregnant woman. Some attention, however, has been focused on the rights of biological unwed fathers in cases of adoption and increasingly in abortion.

RIGHTS AND OBLIGATIONS OF SOCIETY

One of the factors for any society in balancing conflicting values is the question of where to draw the line. In this case, that means under what conditions using which variables will society determine its abortion policy? If society develops a fairly restrictive policy, the argument could be made that some women would be threatened by the continuation of pregnancy, the new child would place great economic and psychological burdens on the family, the mode of existence and the lives of some women would be seriously disrupted, and physically or mentally disabled infants would be born. On the other hand, if the policy permits women to obtain abortion with no restrictions or at least very limited restrictions, the "slippery slope" argument can be brought into the discussion. This argument says that there may be good reasons adduced for doing or not doing something because of what may possibly or predictably follow: What will come to be the case if our society does X? Will this social practice have consequences on other practices? Applied to the abortion situation, the questions develop as follows: If social policy makes abortion available, will this lead society to diminish its reverence for life and possibly to a lessening of its collective instinct for protecting the helpless? Would one such policy lead to other policies affecting the elderly, the mentally ill, and the developmentally disabled? Could such policies push a society into disregarding the life of others who may not be productive or who may be a burden on society, such as chronically ill or elderly people? It is interesting to note that abortion has been legal in Sweden and Japan for many years, and some social scientists say those societies meet their obligations to these vulnerable groups better than the United States does.

In a world as interrelated as our own, some have taken the position that population control has become an overriding problem affecting every society and have suggested abortion as one method to deal with this problem. Using demographic, economic, sociological, and psychological data, population experts have argued for and against abortion as an important means of birth control. The issue can be argued from a moral perspective, and on that basis, some have decided against abortion as a permissible means of population control. The problem of population control can be approached from another perspective. While it is acknowledged that the need for population control is important, specific techniques are not the solution. Rather, it has been shown that improving the economic conditions and the overall well-being of women reduces birth rates, thus reducing or eliminating the need for abortion.

The crux of the ethical dilemma of abortion and the rights and obligations of society can be summarized in two questions. First, does society derive some benefits in legally and socially restricting abortion that override the benefits to the pregnant woman of being able to make her own decisions? This question points out the need to balance the rights and obligations of society as a whole against the rights and obligations of the individual member of that society. Second, what ideals will inform our abortion policy? Will they turn on the definition of what constitutes human life or on the meanings we attach to the conditions—psychological, social, and economic—that are necessary for human life? Is agreement possible? If not, what social policy would work best in a pluralistic democracy?

The moral positions in any pluralistic society tend to reflect many diverse values, which can lead to intolerance of other viewpoints. The most difficult challenge for society and its members is the incommensurability of the positions and the moral passion each side brings to the abortion debate. There is no shared language or understanding of the issues, and there is no common point from which to have dialogue. Militant stances result, and the way we live with each other and each other's different values raises a central ethical question.

Abortion is a societal issue that will not easily go away and, indeed, some argue that it should not go away. The central moral problems in the debate have remained remarkably stable over the years. The personhood argument says that either (a) the fetus lacks personhood and therefore is not entitled to protection against being killed or (b) the fetus is a person and has this entitlement. The bodily support argument says that even if the personhood of the fetus were established, the choice of continuing the pregnancy belongs to the woman whose body is involved in that pregnancy. In the final analysis, how we understand ourselves as a people and how we define membership in this community is the larger concern for our society.

ABORTION AND NURSING

In 1967, the *American Journal of Nursing* (*AJN*) published a paper on abortion that pointed out that as society's views change, the law changes (Hershey, 1967). This reflected the ferment going on in the years just before the Supreme Court decision. At the American Nurses Association (ANA) 1968 convention, the Division of Maternal and Child Health Nursing Practice presented a Statement to Study State Abortion Legislation.[4] The delegates approved this statement with some discussion on whether the organization should take a stand on such a controversial issue that might be misunderstood. They expressed concern over the loose application of abortion laws that could result in serious risks to women and their families and expressed support of movements to examine and modify existing abortion laws. At about the same time, an essay on nurses' attitudes and abortion addressed the issue of personal moral positions and professional obligations (Fonseca, 1968). During the late 1960s and early 1970s, the *AJN* kept its readers abreast of the changes occurring in the state abortion laws and of the changes and nurses' reactions to them in the United Kingdom. In addition, it reported the proceedings of an interdisciplinary panel on abortion. Throughout the early 1970s, the *AJN* reported activities and experiences of individuals and groups concerned with abortion. Occasionally, a paper presenting some aspects of nursing care and abortion appeared. In January 1972, the *Journal* editor said in an editorial on abortion that "the search for moral values is part of what makes one human. Respecting the rights of others in their search also makes one humane" (Schorr, 1972).

In refusing to provide patient care, it has been concluded that nurses may morally refuse a patient care assignment if, and only if, certain conditions are met. One such condition is refusal on religio-moral grounds, when those objections have been made known in advance. No emergency can exist nor can the patient be placed in jeopardy by the refusal. This condition would cover refusal to participate in the act of abortion itself. Whether it covers a refusal to care for the patient before or after the abortion is problematic in light of the ANA Code for Nurses, which states that nurses care for patients regardless of the patient's values and lifestyle. A number of nurses have also addressed the nature of the nurse's duty to care (Brown & Davis, 1990; Frye, 1993).

In a 1992 poll the researchers found a change in the number of nurses (61 percent) who said they would not work in obstetrical and gynecological units performing abortions (Horsley, 1992). If nurses find that because of their values they cannot condone abortion on any grounds, then the likelihood of their being able to care for an abortion patient without exhibiting unkind or even punitive behavior may be diminished. State laws have been enacted in most states that protect the individual who refuses to perform or participate in an abortion because this procedure is contrary to his or her conscience or religious beliefs. Such laws make the violation of this provision by an employer a misdemeanor. Furthermore, these laws indicate that no civil action for negligence or malpractice shall be maintained against a person refusing to perform or participate in an abortion. Every nurse confronted with this situation has both the right and the obligation to obtain information regarding state laws and institution policies on this matter.

A slightly more complicated situation may arise when nurses approve of abortion for certain reasons but not for others, or when they believe abortion should be limited to the first trimester. Some nurses can work with patients admitted for a dilation and curettage procedure, since these abortions occur early in their pregnancies, while these same nurses find it difficult, if not impossible, to work with patients aborted by the saline method, since the fetuses will be further along in development. If the patient's values match the nurses' category of permissible abortion, they should have no real ethical problems in proving care; however, if they do not match, these nurses will need to find a solution to this ethical dilemma in which personal value system and professional obligations conflict. A head nurse or nursing supervisor can play an important role here by discussing the issues with the staff nurse, provided his or her awareness of the ethical dilemma includes the balancing of the rights of the nurse as a person with the obligations of the nurse as a professional.

Perhaps, the most worrisome type of situation arises with nurses who either have given little thought to their ethical position on abortion or in order to maintain their jobs deny to themselves that they harbor resentment toward abortion patients. One can only hope that each nurse will seriously think about his or her beliefs about these issues. It is important for nurses to know where they morally draw the line for what they think is right or wrong, have some understanding of how they reached that conclusion, and realize how it will affect the provision of nursing care.

In the last analysis, the nurse must arrive at a balance between his or her own values and the professional obligations to the patient. In the process of reasoning through the ethical dilemmas involved in abortion, the least that can be hoped for is that the patient will not be abandoned. The most that can be hoped for is that each nurse regards the rights of others as precious, as he or she would want his or her own regarded. Within this complex context, the nurse must engage in critical ethical reflection on the obligations to self, to the patient, to the nursing profession, and to his or her place of employment.

In recent years, numerous sources have become available addressing the ethical issues of abortion. You need to know what ethical positions are being made about the moral status of the embryo in these sources. Not all of them present arguments for both the right of choice and the right to life. But this has been attempted in this chapter.

This chapter ends with an additional and more recently posed ethical dilemma. Should advance nurse practitioners perform abortion services? When you think about these dilemmas, also think about the ANA Code for Nurses and the 1989 ANA Position Paper on Reproductive Health.[5]

CASE STUDY I

Julie is a 17-year-old pregnant teenager who is receiving prenatal care at a nurse-run prenatal clinic. She had a baby last year. She decided to keep the baby with the help of her family, with whom she lives. She has been attending high school and had hoped to graduate next year. However, she dropped out of school recently as she had not been feeling "up to par" with this pregnancy. She works part time as a cashier at a local coffee shop.

You are the nurse practitioner caring for Julie. Julie told you on her first visit that she had been exposed to rubella 3 weeks earlier when her little brother and several of his classmates had "the measles." She is just entering the second trimester. You have explained to Julie and her mother the risks to the fetus from this exposure. Her mother wants her to have an abortion as she already provides most of the care for Julie's child. Julie, however, refuses to have an abortion saying that she loves this baby and is praying the baby should not have been affected.

Suggested Questions for Discussion

1. What are the ethical issues or concerns in this situation?
2. What is the unit of ethical analysis: the fetus, the mother, the grandmother, the family, or society?
3. What are the nurse's obligations, to whom, and why?

CASE STUDY II

Ms. B. recently graduated *magna cum laude* from a very prominent law school. She is married to a very successful architect, Mr. C., and they currently live on the West Coast. They have been waiting to start a family until she completed law school, and she quickly became pregnant after graduation. She is somewhat ambivalent about the pregnancy, but her husband is anxious to start a family.

Ms. B. is offered the very prestigious honor of clerking for a Supreme Court Justice just as she enters her eighth week of pregnancy. This is a lifelong dream come true, and she wants very much to accept this position. However, she realizes it would be impossible to care for a child in the way she and her husband want to while carrying out the demanding work of a Supreme Court Clerk. She now views this pregnancy as a hindrance and wants to undergo an abortion. Her husband would like to have the child. She decides to have an abortion.

Suggested Questions for Discussion

1. What constitutes a legitimate reason for an abortion? Is having a legitimate reason necessary?
2. What are Ms. B.'s rights and Mr. C.'s rights in this situation?
3. What are your moral judgments in this case, and how would they affect your care of Ms. B.?

Notes

1. *Roe v Wade*. 410 US 113 (1973).
2. Guttmacher Institute, Abortion in the United States and the world, www.prb.org/Article/2005 (accessed February 12, 2008).
3. American Medical Association: *22 Transcript* 258, 1871.
4. American Nurses Association: Division of Maternal and Child Health Nursing Practice, Statement to Study State Abortion Legislation 1968.
5. American Nurses Association: Position Paper on Reproductive Health, 1989.

References

American Medical Association. (1967, June). *Proceedings of the House of Delegates*, pp. 40–51.

American Medical Association. (1970, June). *Proceedings of the House of Delegates*, p. 221.

Atwood, M. (1987). *The handmaid's tale*. New York: Ballantine Books.

Brown, J. S., & Davis, A. J. (1990). Ethical issues in refusing to provide patient care. In N. Chaska (Ed.), *The nursing profession: Turning points* (pp. 313–320). St. Louis: CV Mosby.

Fonseca, J. D. (1968). Induced abortion: Nursing attitudes and actions. *American Journal of Nursing, 68*, 1022–1027.

Francome, C. (2004). *Abortion in the USA and UK*. Burlington, VT: Ashgate Publishing Company.

Frye, B. S. (1993). *Abortion. AWHONNS Clinical Issues in Perinatal and Women's Health Nursing, 4*(2), 265–271.

Ginsburg, R. B. (1994). Some thoughts on autonomy and equality in relation to *Roe v Wade*. In L. P. Pojman & F. J. Beckwith (Eds.), *The abortion controversy* (pp. 119–128). Boston: Jones and Bartlett.

Hershey, N. (1967). As society's views change, laws change. *American Journal of Nursing, 67*, 2310–2312.

Horsley, J. (1992). Abortion and nursing: A legal update. *RN, 55*(12), 57–58.

Hull, N. E. H., & Hoffer, P. C. (2001). *Roe v Wade: The abortion rights controversy in American history*. Lawrence, KS: Press of Kansas University.

Landis, J. (Ed.). (2006). *Abortion (History of issues)*. Farmington Hills: Greenhaven Press.

Legge, J. S. (1985). *Abortion policy: An evaluation of the consequences for material and infant health*. New York: SUNY Press.

Riddle, J. M. (1994). *Contraception and abortion from the ancient world to the renaissance*. Cambridge: Harvard University Press.

Riddle, J. M. (1997). *Eve's herbs: A history of contraception and abortion in the East*. Cambridge: Harvard University Press.

Schoen, J. (2005). *Choices and coercion: Birth control, sterilization and abortion in public health and welfare*. Chapel Hill: University North Carolina Press.

Schorr, T. M. (1972). Issues of conscience. *American Journal of Nursing, 72*, 61.

Sherwin, S. (1992). *No longer patient: Feminist ethics and health care*. Philadelphia: Temple University Press.

CHAPTER 8

Dying and Death

INTRODUCTION

Issues surrounding dying and death raise many ethical concerns and questions for nurses, the nursing profession, and the public. Many of these issues evoke our personal feelings of ambiguity or fear about death, but some forms of dying challenge the view that death is the worst thing that can happen to us. Nurses provide care to patients throughout the life span, from before birth to after death. Through the use of sophisticated life-support technology and treatments, the process of dying has often been prolonged in hospitals or nursing homes, where most Americans die and where most nurses are employed. In the face of these facts, it is not always clear that ethical principles such as respect for persons or the non infliction of harm have been considered in clinical practice involving the dying patient.

Over the last several decades, we have encountered troubling questions about when death actually occurs, the quality of life, the sanctity of life, do-not-resuscitate orders, disclosure of terminal diagnoses to patients, and the individual's right to die with dignity, including the right to receive active assistance in dying from health professionals. There are other questions as well. How should the interests of the individual patient, the family, health care professionals, and the community be weighed in making a decision about a congenitally deformed infant, who will die without a sequence of painful surgical interventions and the use of costly medical resources? Who should decide?

Does a patient or a family have the right to choose to "do everything" clinically when such a treatment is futile and will not extend the patient's life? What is futile? How do we know?

Does an individual have the right to choose death? Is there a moral difference between letting a person die and taking an action to hasten death? When, if ever, should life-sustaining treatment be withheld from patients who are unable to make this decision themselves? The implications of these questions are far-reaching and demand a thoughtful response from health care professionals, patients, families, the community, and society.

When the now famous 1976 landmark Quinlan case in New Jersey came to public attention through the mass media, it served to refocus some of these questions for health professionals, for other professions (such as law and theology), and for the entire nation. More recently in 2005, Terri Schiavo, a 41-year-old woman, had her feeding tube removed and was allowed to die after a lengthy legal battle between her parents, who argued that Terri was conscious, and her husband/guardian, who in 1998 filed a petition in the court for this action. Terri had collapsed in 1990 and by 1998 had been diagnosed in persistent vegetative state. This tragedy, reported extensively in the media, had members of the U.S. Congress taking public positions on the ethical and clinical actions necessary, without being directly involved (Diesser, 2005). Even the Pope felt compelled to comment on this live case. Such a situation shows the need for all adults to have an advance directive, but this is often not the case since this document forces us to face the reality of our mortality. There is a growing trend in court decisions to recognize a right of the patient, under certain circumstances, to have medical food and fluid withheld.

These types of situations poignantly illustrate the burdens placed on nurses by decisions made by others but which nurses are expected to implement. Importantly, it is the clinical areas of palliative care where nurses have made a difference in the options available to patients and their families, such as the development of hospice care, and in initiating changes in the decision-making process related to development of guidelines for orders not to resuscitate. Nurses are the mainstay in comfort care for the dying.

The ethical, legal, medical, social, cultural, psychological, and economic factors to be considered in near-death interventions (or decisions not to intervene) reflect individual, family, community, and professional values, and these factors must arbitrate between and among these values. The numbers and kinds of factors, including values and clinical facts, intersecting in each situation serve to further muddy the waters of decision making. The immediate decision is often fraught with numerous distant implications, not the least of which includes social policy. But, before a discussion of end-of-life ethics, we would be well advised to reflect on the end of life, per se.

In this chapter, different ethical view points will be discussed. This indicates that, due to cultural, religious, and other factors, not all people in the United States agree on what to do about the ethical issues surrounding dying and death. This is a major topic found in bioethics and nursing ethics journals and in the health professional literature in general.

DETERMINING WHEN SOMEONE IS DYING OR DEAD

The definition of the word "dead" as commonly used ranges on a continuum from having ended existence as a living or growing thing, to being without power to move, feel, or respond, to being incapable of feeling of or not being stirred emotionally or intellectually. Both a process and an event are implied in these various notions of the word "dead."

Tolstoy's novel, *The Death of Ivan Ilyich*, offers a telling description of the social, psychological, and physical aspects of death as a process for the individual and family (Tolstoy, 1967). These varied aspects of "death" and "dead" raise all the questions mentioned previously and increase the complexity for those who make decisions about whether or not respiratory support equipment should be discontinued or extraordinary measures begun for a particular individual.

Traditionally, the physician made the decisions concerning the dying patient. Not so many years ago, these decisions involved primarily the provision of comfort and reassurance for the patient and family. With the more recent trend toward "death with dignity" the patient is or should also be involved in the choices of how to live while dying, the use of drugs to relieve pain, and the decision not to use medical measures that do not prolong a life of quality or promote a cure. Three possible approaches for the physician have been identified:

1. Using all possible means, including extraordinary measures to keep the patient alive
2. Discontinuing extraordinary measures but continuing ordinary means
3. Taking some active steps to intentionally hasten the individual's death

In making such decisions, factors taken into account are the determination of what is extraordinary or burdensome, versus ordinary or beneficial for a particular patient, and whether it refers to experimental drugs, complicated life-maintaining equipment, or antibiotics. (Though they are still commonly used in clinical settings, the terms "ordinary" and "extraordinary" have largely fallen into disuse among ethicists.) These decisions also raise moral questions about which factors *ought* to figure in the decision-making process. For example, patients may be perceived as being more valuable to the living if they can be declared dead so that organs or tissues from their body can be used to benefit others. Some would see this action as using one person primarily as a means to prolonging or improving another's life. Some patients and families view this as doing good since it benefits others. In addition to these factors, a very basic question is whether one has the right to die and, if so, under what circumstances?

Fear that a *right to die*, which involves patient choice in continuing or discontinuing treatment, may lead to a *duty to die*, without patient choice, so as to lessen the social and economic burden placed on families and society.

While the definitions of death give clues about the process of death, they do not help to determine the moment of death. In contemporary health care, the moment of death is often obscured the use of ventilators, balloon pumps, or other life-sustaining technologies that change biometric readings and can keep the patient in vegetative state for some time. A question that must be raised in these discussions is whether there is more to life than biological life. Obviously, biological life is necessary to life and living, but the question that remains is whether biological life is the whole of human life.

Ethics and Law

The determination of death clearly demonstrates the interaction of ethics and the law. Some states have legislated a definition of death based on ordinary standards of medical practice, including loss of spontaneous brain function. Other states have passed legislation that includes brain-death criteria. Both the clinical criteria and the statutes provide guidelines and a process for determining that biological death has occurred. The Uniform Declaration of Death Act of 1980 gives two options for determining death: (a) irreversible cessation of circulation and respiratory function, referred to as cardiopulmonary death and (b) irreversible cessation of all functions of the brain, referred to as brain death (Butts & Rich, 2005). Since brain functions cease when there has been cardiopulmonary cessation, brain death is an alternative way to *measure* that cardiopulmonary cessation has occurred. That is, brain death is not a new definition of death but rather an alternative way of measuring that death has occurred.

To some extent, the process of dying is partially controlled today by individuals themselves in the choices they make about the use of or refusal to use available technologies or treatments. With this relative control over the time of death comes the necessity to think very carefully about who should be involved in making decisions relating to this control, and what elements are important in the decision-making process.

Death can be delayed or prevented with the use of sophisticated technologies. Should these technologies be used simply because they are available? The ethical issues involved in the *technological imperative* ask whether just because technology is available, must it always be used. Should elderly comatose patients be taken thrice a week for dialysis from a nursing home to a renal dialysis center? A patient-centered ethic requires that the individual patient remains the center of the decisions, but what exactly does this mean? All of these issues and questions pivot on questions about the sanctity of life and the quality of life when dying is prolonged through medical and nursing interventions. Discussions of euthanasia follow closely on the discussions of the quality of life when dying is prolonged through the use of technology.

EUTHANASIA: THE GOOD DEATH

The word *euthanasia*, from the Greek, means good death. Is death ever preferable to life? Is there a moral difference between letting die and hastening death, in light of the moral law that says one should not kill? At present, there are mixed responses to these questions. The best interests for a particular patient in a specific situation should stand at the center of these responses, and this must be distinguished from the interests of the provider, social institutions, and society. The following discussion focuses primarily on the dying adult patient and on ethical (as distinct from religious) considerations per se.

In attempting to help patients attain a good death, the following questions serve as a first step.

1. Who decides? The physician, guardian, patient, family member, clergyperson, or a committee or some combination of these?
2. For whom does one decide? Oneself, another person for whom one is acting as a proxy, or others?
3. What additional criteria are used (e.g., psychological, religious, economic, and/or social) after the medical status of the patient has been established?
4. What degree of consent is required of the patient? In this regard, patients fall into four categories: (a) brain-dead adults or minors, (b) terminally ill competent adults, (c) terminally ill incompetent adults, and (d) minors. The way of determining what to do differs in each of these cases.

Decision making should also consider the moral principles involved: respect for the patient's autonomy or best interests, the obligation to do no harm, and the requirement to tell the truth. Are these being affirmed or negated by particular alternatives proposed? Some believe that euthanasia should be considered only in relation to those who have voluntarily expressed the desire to die, and this is commonly called voluntary euthanasia. This position eliminates newborns and infants from its consideration. It also excludes those individuals on life-support and the elderly with severe senile dementia who are unable to participate in decision making. An advance directive could help families and health professionals in such situations.

One position says that newborns in certain circumstances, such as severely deformed or extremely premature newborns, should be allowed to die by withdrawing or withholding treatment. These decisions should be made by parents with the assistance of professional advisors, usually physicians, since the parents are most familiar with the human complexities of their situation. In past years, when parental decisions for nontreatment of infants have been brought to the courts, most court decisions have required that treatment be given. These decisions make it clear that there has been a general legal duty to treat a child. These opposing views again reflect the complexity and conflict that exist when we attempt to answer the ethical questions surrounding dying and death.

Decision makers have a continuum of interventions for decision making ranging from an anti-euthanasia absolutist position based on an understanding of the *sanctity of life* to an equally absolutist proeuthanasia view based on notions of an inadequate *quality of life*, or on a supposed absolute right to decide. The absolutist anti-euthanasia position commits one to vigorous treatment to preserve life at any and all costs, referred to as *vitalism*, and is not in accord with a general understanding of the sanctity of life principle. More moderate positions require the use of non burdensome treatments, without necessarily requiring the use of what have been called heroic measures. There is difficulty in determining exactly what constitutes (and who decides what constitutes) non burdensomeness and heroics. If we follow the general norm that the patient's values and decisions determine his or her own care, what constitutes burdensomeness becomes particularly difficult to determine when the patient cannot express the degree of burden that he or she feels.

Earlier, there was a generalized agreement, and many defined *ordinary (non-burdensome)* means of preserving life to include all medicines, treatments, and surgical procedures that offer reasonable hope of benefit to a patient and that could be obtained and used without excessive pain, expense, or other inconveniences. *Extraordinary* (or *burdensome*) means are those that are very costly, unusual, difficult, or dangerous, or do *not* offer a reasonable hope of benefit to the patient. These determinations may vary in a large teaching hospital from the ones made in a small community hospital or in another setting where the dying individual is placed. What may be considered ordinary or non-burdensome treatment to or for one patient may be considered extraordinary or burdensome to or for another—for example, the use of antibiotics for a patient with pneumonia only as opposed to the use of antibiotics for treating pneumonia in the patient who has terminal cancer with metastases to the brain and liver.

Some regard withdrawal of treatment to let the patient die as a form of passive euthanasia, while others maintain that it is the intent (i.e., the patient's death is intended) rather than the withdrawal of treatment itself that determines whether or not euthanasia is involved. In letting die, treatment that offers no hope of recovery and serves only to prolong dying is withheld or ongoing treatment withdrawn, with or without the consent of the patient. The withdrawal of treatment to allow a patient to die is still an ethically controversial topic for some health professionals even though it has received ample attention in the ethical and clinical literature, to the point of being considered a settled question by many though not all.

Active and Passive Euthanasia

Active euthanasia includes such actions as giving patients the means to kill themselves (assisted suicide) or directly bringing about the patient's death with or without consent, for instance, through a lethal injection of potassium chloride.

Do patients have the right to control their dying, and if so where does this right of patients to control their own dying fit into our consideration of euthanasia? Do individuals have the right to die or even to kill themselves in a hospital historically committed to preserving life? Can a patient refuse potentially beneficial life-saving treatment? Do health professionals have an obligation to agree to this patient's decision and participate in it?

There is no provision in the law that compels a competent person to seek medical care, except when the illness is a threat to public health or safety—for example, with a communicable disease. In several legal cases, the hospital and the attending physician were not required to perform surgery or give transfusions against the patient's will. There have been contradictory legal findings in various cases, where individuals refused life-saving blood transfusions because of religious beliefs. In 1977, the Massachusetts Supreme Court decided in the famous *Saikewicz* case that the courts should most appropriately make decisions about nontreatment for those incompetent to make their own decisions. This court also affirmed that all patients have the right to refuse life-sustaining treatment that will not cure the illness or preserve life (Carroll, 1978).

In the early 1980s, the U.S. President appointed a commission to investigate several major ethical issues. That commission, called the President's Commission for the Study of Ethical Problems in Medicine and Biomedical and Behavioral Research, issued two reports entitled *Defining Death* and *Deciding to Forego Life-Sustaining Treatment*. In the latter report, the President's Commission maintained that

> Nothing in current law precludes ethically sound decision making. Neither criminal nor civil law—if properly interpreted and applied—forces patients to undergo procedures that will increase their suffering when they wish to avoid this by foregoing life-sustaining treatment.

The commission further held that

> The distinction between failing to initiate and stopping therapy—that is, withholding versus withdrawing treatment—is not itself of moral [or legal] importance. A justification that is adequate for not commencing a treatment is also sufficient for ceasing it. (President's Commission for the Study, 1983)

Life-sustaining treatment may be withheld, or may be withdrawn, when it is against the patient's wishes, provided that the patient is fully informed and freely consenting; it may be withheld or withdrawn when it will or has begun to harm the patient; or when it is not now or projected to benefit the patient.

Thus, for the most part, ethicists have agreed that when life-sustaining treatment will constitute a violation of the patient's dignity, humanity, well-being, or integrity, it need not be given or continued. This has become a settled issue to a very large extent. One area of concern that has yet to be fully resolved is the administration of food and fluid, particularly by medical means.

In using the term *euthanasia*, some authors make a distinction between mercy killing or active euthanasia and allowing people to die or passive euthanasia. They claim that one is an act of commission, while the other, an act of omission. A further distinction is made between voluntary (with patient permission) and involuntary (without patient permission) euthanasia. Other authors define euthanasia as any act by another person that results in *intentionally* bringing about death, whether it is an act of omission or commission. Treatment withdrawal without intent to bring about death does not, therefore, constitute passive euthanasia. It has also been argued that there is no ethical distinction between active and passive euthanasia because the end result, death of the patient, is the same. Acts of omission are seen as not interfering with the natural process of dying, where euthanasia-as-mercy-killing is seen as inducing death. Another distinction is that the right to die is associated only with the individual, while euthanasia demands that someone else intervenes to induce, or assists in inducing, death. This raises the question as to whether society or any of its members should accept such an obligation.

While in the Netherlands both the social consensus and the law condone active euthanasia, in the United States, there have been some serious gaps in the law for dealing with the broad issue of euthanasia (Cohen-Almagor, 2004). Euthanasia has been regarded as a form of homicide, and patient consent or request for euthanasia is not legally acceptable as a defense. The law has taken into account whether the situation involves an act or failure to act. To some extent, the law does make a distinction between active and passive euthanasia. No case in the Anglo-American law has been reported in which a physician was convicted of murder or manslaughter for having withdrawn treatment to end the suffering of a patient. This tradition seems to consider intent of the physician as the defining criterion.

Several different ethical viewpoints on euthanasia are significant to the nurse, other health professionals, and society, seeking to articulate an ethical position on euthanasia. One position, sometimes called the new morality, supports a value system that puts humanness, human dignity, and personal integrity above biological life and functions. This position arises from the belief that the core of humanness lies in the rational faculty, that is, in one's ability or potential to be rational. What counts as an ethically right action is whether or not human needs come first. The ethical defense is that euthanasia reduces suffering and helps the patient die rather than prolonging a slow, painful, dehumanizing death. This position holds the value that death is not the worst thing that can happen to an individual. Both Eastern and Western religious traditions generally agree that one is not morally obligated to preserve life in all cases. For example, the Roman Catholic position says that it is not necessary to use extraordinary means to prolong life for the terminally ill person.

One objection in the United States to euthanasia is that the same thing will happen as happened in Nazi Germany. This is the *slippery slope* or *wedge* argument that claims if beneficent euthanasia, a kindly act, can be ethically justified, then euthanasia for other and possibly unethical purposes—down the slippery slope—may be practiced and justified. This kind of thinking ignores the fact that the Nazis engaged in genocide and killing for ideological reasons, *not* mercy killing in the sense of a merciful act of kindness. On the other hand, one should not ignore the findings of an earlier classic study in which a select group of U.S. university students was asked a variety of questions related to euthanasia and was also asked to suggest a final solution to problems of overpopulation and misery. Over half of the respondents said that society should get rid of unfit persons as a final solution (Mansson, 1972).

It may be more difficult to ethically justify letting a terminally ill person die a slow, dehumanized death than not letting him or her die sooner. The practice of euthanasia-as-merciful-killing implies compassion on the part of the agent and society. Others do not agree, because killing for them has always had evil characteristics, even when killing is in self-defense.

In considering whether or not suffering justifies killing human life, the principle of proportionate good and the Doctrine of Double Effect may be used. The principle of proportionate good means balancing the benefits and harms of an action for the suffering individual. The ethical debate over palliative sedation is the differentiation between sedation for intractable pain and for euthanasia. Health professionals have the ethical obligation to extend life and also to relieve pain. When a patient is terminally ill and near death, the relief of pain ethically outweighs extending life for most practitioners. The Doctrine of Double Effect comes from Roman Catholic theology and is helpful in situations where it is impossible to avoid harmful effects. This doctrine makes the distinction between an intended effect and an unintended effect of an intervention. Intentionally causing death is unacceptable according to this position, but giving high doses of medications to relieve pain is acceptable even if the resulting death is foreseen (McIntyre, 2004). This principle is in line with a quality of life ethic that says that human dignity is important and a good death is more humane than a protracted painful one.

In the face of continuing debate by proponents of active euthanasia and opponents of it, the ethic of obligation suggests the following kinds of care for patients who are considered to be imminently dying:

1. The relief of pain
2. The relief of suffering
3. Respect for the right of an individual to refuse treatment
4. Universal provision of health care in the sense that individuals and families would not have to bear the burden of catastrophic medical care alone.

Decisions Not to Resuscitate and Advance Directives

Regarding the decision not to resuscitate, many in the health professions and the general public believe that this decision is fully compatible with respect for the intrinsic value of human life. Not to resuscitate under specific circumstances can be seen as a refusal to attempt to control life and death further through the use of technology.

Further efforts to clarify the position of individuals and society on the right to die with dignity are found in the development of advance directives, which include the *Living Will,* the *Durable Power of Attorney for Health Care (DPAHC)*, and the emerging *Physician Orders for Life-Sustaining Treatment* (POLST). These are documents in which competent adults can indicate their end-of-life wishes and values. People can change their minds at any time and replace an advance directive with a new one. The Living Will prepared by the organization Concern for Dying was a model for death with dignity bills introduced into state legislatures in the early stages of this legislation.

The landmark Natural Death Act (1976) in California (its living will legislation) recognized the rights of adults to prepare written instructions authorizing their physicians to withhold or withdraw life-sustaining procedures in specified circumstances of terminal illness (California Natural Death Act, 1976). A major purpose of the original bill was to settle a number of legal issues concerned with professional liability and insurance coverage. This Act relieved physicians, health facilities, and other licensed health professionals of civil liability for carrying out directives as defined in the bill. The bill declared that death resulting from carrying out a directive does not constitute suicide, thus resolving this issue in relation to insurance policies as well. Although this legislation provided answers and guidelines for some problems, people recognized that public policy of this import raises a host of additional issues for interpretation.

In addition to the Living Will, a number of states have provisions for designating a DPAHC. Though the legislation varies across states, the DPAHC allows adults to designate another individual (and an alternate) as decision maker for health care decisions when the person cannot make his or her own decisions. Such documents allow for this power of attorney to be given to any adult including a nonfamily member. Some forms of the DPAHC allow the person to specify the sorts of treatments that would or would not be acceptable at the end of life. For the person who holds the power of attorney (emphasis is on *power*; the person need not be a lawyer), his or her decisions have the force of the patient's own decisions and cannot be challenged unless they appear to be clearly contrary to the patient's own wishes. In 1991, the Patient Self-Determination Act became law. Congress passed this law as the first federal legislation to ensure that hospitals and other health care facilities inform patients regarding their rights under state law. In addition, patients were to be informed about institutional policies to accept or refuse medical treatment and their right to have an advance directive. In some health care institutions, nurses are the ones who discuss these issues with patients and their families.[2]

The discussion of active euthanasia and passive euthanasia in the earlier sections of this chapter focused primarily on adult patients. These issues were mentioned only briefly in relation to severely deformed newborns and children with terminal illness. Many of the same issues and questions involving adults apply to children and newborns. A basic difference with children and infants concerns who should make what decisions. The physician? The parents? The older child? One concern is whether or not a society should even consider the nontreatment option for children. What are the implications for individuals and the human community as to the value of life? Some see this as infanticide; others see it as a quality-of-life issue. There are other special issues arising in relation to the death of young children—for example, the legal standing of the rights of children, the status of parental rights, and the obligations of adults to prevent suffering in children. All of these concerns are still raised whenever severely deformed infants and terminally ill children receive care. What are ordinary and extraordinary measures in a newborn intensive care unit? Does the definition depend on the locally available technology? Do health professionals have obligations to always use the technology available, without thinking about how lives are affected by it now and in the foreseeable future (Catlin, 2006)?

In discussions of nontreatment of newborns with birth defects, some have said that the current haphazard, arbitrary patterns of selection for nontreatment will probably continue unless substantive and procedural criteria are developed as guidelines for decision making. The National Association of Neonatal Nurses has developed position statements on numerous ethical issues faced by nurses caring for vulnerable newborn infants (National Association of Neonatal Nurses, 2006). Importantly, the Resolve Through Sharing Bereavement program has been established to help those involved in these difficult decisions surrounding the death of a child (Resolve Through Sharing, 2008).

In summary, this overview of selected issues and complexities of decision making related to euthanasia, death, and dying does not provide us with any ready-made answers. What it does do is give the reader some idea of directions taken by individuals, institutions, and society in seeking ways to make more ethically appropriate decisions when the patient is dying.

SUICIDE AND ASSISTED SUICIDE AS AN ETHICAL DILEMMA

Suicide, a major leading cause of death in the United States, has been seen variously as an affirmation of life, a denial of life, and a questioning of life. The traditional religious teachings of the Western religions have historically condemned all intentional acts of self-destruction. Though it is all too simple a reduction of their position, traditionally Western theologies have regarded life as a gift of God, belonging to God, but given to humankind for its stewardship. Suicide, then, has been seen as a usurpation of God's authority, thus as sin, because it involves the claim that one's life is one's own (and not belonging to God) to do with as one pleases.

The philosopher Kant, who separated religion and ethics, said that humans rightfully do not have the power of disposal of their own bodies. One can treat one's body as one chooses only in relation to self-preservation (Kant, 1976). These traditional religious and philosophical views are being challenged in today's society. Realizing that suicide often occurs when a person is depressed, despondent, or under duress, and thus less than fully voluntary, the Act of 1961 declared that suicide should not any longer be regarded as a *criminal* act.[3]

If one believes that it is permissible to commit suicide, then it is useful to distinguish between rational and nonrational suicide. Rational suicide may be ascribed to those rational persons suffering from a terminal disease and who understand the consequences of their act, exercise their self-determination. However, most persons who commit suicide are not terminally ill but suffer from clinically recognizable psychiatric illnesses and have sought help from physicians. These are cases of nonrational suicide, and health providers have an obligation to do good by not allowing patients to harm themselves.

More recently, the debate has focused on assisted suicide, which means that under certain circumstances people who are severely ill, near death, and who wish to commit suicide should receive help to die from their physicians. Laws exist in the Netherlands, Uruguay, Switzerland, Peru, Japan, and Germany, but not the United States, except in Oregon, that such assistance from the physician. However, fearful of a slippery slope situation, those who support physician-assisted suicide say that this group of patients must be considered separately from the lonely, the elderly, and the physically handicapped, who may also seek to commit suicide and ask another's assistance.

The individual's right to self-determination is a basic consideration in the discussion of the ethical dimensions of suicide and assisted suicide. There are positions at both ends of the continuum that range from the position that individuals have the right to self-determination and that they should retain this right even if they are considered by some to be potentially dangerous or suicidal to the other view that health professionals have the obligation to support the desire for life that may exist such as individuals with terminal illness. Other major arguments against suicide are that it is a crime against society, a cowardly act, a violation of one's duty to God, unnatural, an insult to human dignity, and cruel because it inflicts pain upon one's family and friends.

Arguments have been made that suicide may be ethically justifiable under certain conditions. These arguments include the idea that no rational morality would require that certain lives be continued in the face of disastrous accidents of birth or illnesses where there are no effective remedial measures. Another argument is that no social morality can be equally binding on everyone in society unless there is more equality in distributing the necessities of life such as health care. This is the ethical principle of justice as fairness that promotes a more equal distribution of society's benefits and harms. The obligation to provide a more just society in which all can live well and die peacefully may rest with those who say that one should not commit suicide.

In summary, suicide and assisted suicide are still controversial topics in our society and raise many profound ethical questions for the health professional about the individual's right to self-determination vis-à-vis the right of the human community to preserve itself. Assisted suicide raises profound questions about the aims of the health sciences and the obligations of health professionals to patients and redefines what historically has been considered as good and harmful in the relationship with patients.

FURTHER THOUGHTS FOR NURSING PRACTICE

The nursing literature in the recent past has focused primarily on attitudes toward death and dying patients; the depersonalized, institutionalized dying process; and the nurse's personal experiences with dying patients and their families. Now, much more is written on the ethical dilemmas faced by nurses caring for dying patients and their families.

Nurses should examine, individually and collectively, their own values in relation to death, quality of life, the needs of the dying patient, and such moral principles as self-determination for the dying patient, the bases of respect for the person, the obligation to do no harm, distributive justice, and the caring dimensions of the nurse–patient relationship.

One of the nurse's *legal* responsibilities is to follow medical orders. An issue that arises for nurses is that they do not always have written orders on which to rely. For example, decisions will be made by nurses for specific patients if they have a cardiac arrest and only verbal no-code orders exist. It is generally understood that if there is no written orders for no-code and a patient experiences cardiac arrest, the nurse must code the patient.

Physicians have the primary ethical and legal obligation to explore the implications of the no-code decision with the patient and family, but the initial judgment should be discussed with the other physicians, nurses, and any others directly involved with the patient's care. This provides an opportunity for nurses to add their observations and assessment of a patient to that of others in the decision-making process and *caring* for the dying patient. It is the responsibility of the physician not only to actually record the order not to resuscitate but also to convey the meaning of this order for a particular patient to medical, nursing, and other appropriate staff members. Nurses are in a key position to notify the physician if the patient's condition changes.

Nurses are involved in the emotional support needed by the patient's family as they are often the most constant resource for them. Some specific needs of these relatives are to be with the dying person, to be helpful to the dying person, to be assured of the comfort of the dying person, to be informed of the patient's condition, to be informed of impending death, to be able to express emotions, to have the comfort and support of other family members, and to have acceptance, support, and comfort from health professionals. Spouses often note that nurses had been helpful to their dying mates but may be perceived as being too busy to help the families. Nurses can be facilitators for meeting most of these needs, even in intensive care settings, by making themselves available to families. This is not without strain and tension for the nurse.

An important question is whether nursing administration has a moral obligation to provide support systems for nursing staff caring for critically ill and dying patients. Some institutions already provide such support for nurses and physicians through psychologists or chaplains. Nurses can also initiate collaborative efforts with others, such as chaplains and social workers, to meet the needs of families of dying patients.

Clinical ethics committees often discuss issues of care for the dying. These discussions can fall into two categories: those from the participants' point of view and those from the administrative perspective. Nurses and physicians are usually in the first group—that is, they often identify with the patient and what they assume to be in the best interests of the patient. The second perspective views the dying patient as a managerial problem and is more concerned with the use of hospital resources. Problems are implicit in both of these viewpoints. The participant's perspective in advocating death with dignity and the rights of patients to refuse treatment can ignore when and under what conditions patients might choose death. Health professionals must also guard against imposing their own values on patients and families. The administrative viewpoint, concerned with efficient use of resources and the equality of treatment for all patients, can ignore the diversity of individual patient needs. With the development of managed care, these two perspectives, which can conflict, become even more important to examine from an ethical perspective.

Some have taken the position that in disagreements between these viewpoints, questions should be resolved as *patient* policy questions, not as hospital or public policy questions, such as those concerning limited beds or other limited hospital resources. The potential danger that exists is that more decisions will be based on economic considerations or on a utilitarian ethic that considers only the common good as the determinant in decision making. In light of this, one needs to also discuss the moral principles of doing no harm, justice as equal treatment, and respect for values of patients and families, with both the common good and individual needs considered.

Nursing emphasizes the importance of *caring* for dying patients beyond the point where life can be preserved. Nurses and other health professionals are healers and menders of patients; however, in caring for patients, some dimensions of the patient's life are beyond the professional's appropriate concern. These areas are more appropriate to the concern and attention of the family or the patient's significant others because these persons are most intimately involved with the patient. Difficult decision making arises when nurses care for an individual who does not have family or significant others when particular problems occur, and when it is inappropriate for health professionals to intervene. This becomes a particularly sensitive issue when the patient is unable to make these decisions; in such a situation, legal intervention may be necessary to secure a guardian or a conservator.

It is a duty for one to never abandon *care*. In caring for the dying person, one may eventually cease doing what was once called for and begin to do what is now required in the individual situation. This does not mean that one is required to assist the dying process, but that one must assure the person that she or he is not alone and that others are aware of this dying and will be there during this time. Recall the needs and concerns of family members of dying persons mentioned earlier.

These caring values and practices are clearly demonstrated in the hospice movement where death is neither hastened nor prolonged. It has been suggested that we could formulate a moral rule that the *only* circumstance in which positive action might be taken to hasten a person's death is if there is the kind of prolonged dying where it is medically impossible to control the individual's pain or other distressing symptoms. Physician-assisted suicide and active euthanasia could result from such a formulation. The nurse, through close contact in caring for the patient and managing control of symptoms, may be the first to see that this situation has been reached by a particular patient. It becomes imperative for the nurse to communicate this to the patient's physician. The ethic and practice of allowing to die, recognized by most health professionals, still leaves the question as to whether physicians can take positive action to hasten death without weakening medicine's life-saving ethic. It must also be noted that actively helping a patient to die is not an acceptable solution to poor symptom control. It is important to realize that the clinical definition of pain is often limited to concerns for physical pain. But there is also psychological pain that is more akin to suffering. Physical pain can often be controlled, while psychological pain in some instances may be beyond the reach of health professionals. In concert with others, such as family members or a religious counselor, health professionals can attempt to help patients ease their suffering.

As far back as 1971, a study of nurses' feelings about euthanasia was conducted (Brown, Thompson, Bulger, & Laws, 1971). The findings indicated that nurses heard requests for positive or direct euthanasia from terminally ill patients and their families more frequently than did physicians. The underlying assumption was that this was a consequence of the fact that nurses have more interaction with the patient and family than do physicians. More nurses were uncomfortable when physicians did not let patients, irretrievably dying, die than when the physician did follow this ethic. Nurses generally demonstrated more desire than physicians for social changes, such as legislation, to allow euthanasia. These nurses said that the patient has a right to maintain control and make decisions about the end of his or her life and way of dying. More nurses than physicians supported the concept of using a committee or a board for resolving difficult philosophical decisions about questions of euthanasia.

Nursing, as a profession, has articulated an ethic of care for the dying. In the recent past, a moral distinction has been made between acts that *permit* death and acts that cause death. According to this ethic, the compassion and freedom of the nurse are increased as the nurse cares for an irreversibly ill patient who has the freedom to refuse interventions that only prolong the dying process and to make choices such as how to live while dying. This ethic adheres to the universal commandment "thou shalt not kill" and stands in the ethical tradition of principle-based ethics and notions of obligations. Nurses can help patients and families to look at hospice or hospice-like options for care, such as care at home when appropriate support is available. Nurses need to be particularly sensitive to families when home care is not a viable choice. There have been situations where home care has been inappropriately imposed on families by well-meaning health professionals. The major focus should be on preserving the life and values of the human community, with mercy and compassion for the individual.

Some Final Comments

Obviously, our society has not yet reached a consensus on this ethical issue. As there may be recognized conflict between the authority and the autonomy of the health professionals and that of the patient, patients need someone outside of this conflict who represents their interests. Health professionals have traditionally adhered to the ethic that says one should do everything one can to preserve life. Death has been seen as the failure of medical technology and knowledge. Now there is a growing division between those who support the patient's right to die and those who do not see this as a right and who give more weight to the health professional's obligation to treat. With the dying patient, what we mean by treatment needs to be examined and perhaps reconceptualized.

The philosophy of the hospice movement provides a starting point for nurses confronted with a patient and family who want a respirator turned off or do not want heroic measures instituted. The Dying Person's Bill of Rights offers another framework for discussions and decision making about ethical issues in the care of the dying person, whether an adult or a child. *The Dying Person's Bill of Rights* includes such ideas as rights to treatment as a living human being until death, maintenance of a sense of hopefulness, expression of one's own feelings and emotions about approaching death, participation in decisions concerning one's care, freedom from pain, the right not to die alone, the right to have one's questions answered honestly without deception, the right to maintain one's individuality, and the right to be cared for by caring, sensitive, and knowledgeable people. These rights parallel many of the needs identified by families of dying patients. The last right (to be cared for by caring, sensitive, and knowledgeable people) implies that these people, including nurses, have deliberated and continue to consider the ethical dimensions of questions posed by the availability of technologies that may or may not be used to maintain life.

To focus primarily on a patient-centered ethic, as has been done in this section, is not to ignore the hospital policy and public policy issues that have arisen in connection with society's priorities for health and illness and allocation of finite resources. Health policy often directs what we can and cannot do clinically. This important topic is discussed in another chapter.

Advance directives, hospital and nursing home guidelines for orders not to resuscitate, and court and legislative actions are significant steps in resolving some of the ethical dilemmas concerning dying and death. Nurses should take the opportunities to articulate and think through positions on these dilemmas that confront them as individuals and professions. Ethics rounds, courses in basic nursing education, and continuing education efforts in patient care ethics provide forums for doing this within the nursing community and with other health disciplines. The American Nurses Association Center for Ethics and Human Rights provides consultation and serves as a clearinghouse on ethics materials.

Nursing efforts in truly caring for the terminally ill and dying patient have made positive differences at the individual level of care and at the institutional policy level that are reflections of respect for persons. Concerns focus primarily on *how* to treat the dying patient rather than on whether one should treat or not. While futility of treatment has become a major topic in medicine, it is not central to nursing because nurses provide care to patients until they die and even after death (Taylor, 1995). This latter circumstance involves organ donation. Some believe there is a need for mandated choice in which adults are required to consider organ donation and document their decision. These wishes would be legally binding, as opposed to current policy that allows a patient's wishes to be overruled by the family (Saver, 2008).

Since this book was first published in 1978, palliative care has become more central in nursing education and practice. Nurses have explored research topics of pain management and other aspects of caring for dying patients (Ferrell & Covie, 2005). Clinically, many nurses are now better prepared to give competent care because of these changes. Nurse ethicists have taken a major interest in the ethics of dying and death because nursing care always has something to benefit patients and help them attain a good, humane death (Ferrell & Covie, 2008; Matzo, 2006).

CASE STUDY I

You are a hospice nurse who has been caring for Mr. J. for the past 4 months. He is dying of AIDS. He is a high school English teacher, and literature has been the love of his life. He has been doing reasonably well until the last 6 weeks. He now has recurrent cytomegalovirus attacks and is losing his vision. His T-cell count is less than 15.

You have had a very warm relationship, and he has freely shared his hopes, fears, and concerns about his illness. On your visit today, he tells you how much he misses being able to read, and how full his life has been, and that he wants to die. You explore with him how you could make him more comfortable and he says "I'm just tired of this disease, I don't want anymore surprises. It's time to see what comes next. I've planned my farewell for Thursday; some friends are coming to read my favorite poetry. I'd really like you to be here."

Suggested Questions for Discussion

1. What will you do? What motivates your decision?
2. How would you articulate your reasoning to your colleagues?
3. What is the nature of your responsibility to Mr. J.—ethically, legally, and personally? What are the origins of these responsibilities? Are there limits to these responsibilities?

CASE STUDY II

You are a new grad of six months working the night shift on a small cancer unit. There are two RNs on this unit and you are the more senior. Mr. V. has been in and out of this unit several times over the last few months. He has liver cancer and has gone through several episodes of chemotherapy. His last admission, however, was for an unsuccessful suicide attempt. At the time, you learned that he had made several such attempts in the last few weeks.

Mr. V. recently joined the hospice program. His current admission is for pain control, and the orders are to start a morphine drip to be titrated for pain. The only set parameters are to decrease the drip for respirations less than 4 per minute. Mr. V. requests that the drip be increased several times during your shift. Even though he does not appear to be in any discomfort, you accept his assessment and increase the drip. His wife has been staying with him since his admission. On a routine check, you note that his respirations are now 4 per minute and he is unarousable. You turn off the drip, telling the wife that you will turn it back on if he arouses at all or shows any signs of being in pain but that his respirations are dangerously low. After about an hour, he begins to arouse and you resume the drip at a lower level. After about 10 more minutes, Mr. V. wakes up and is furious with you, accusing you of bringing him back from death. "I have a do-not-resuscitate order; you are supposed to let me die." You reply that you did not bring him back; you stopped pushing him toward death.

Suggested Questions for Discussion

1. How do you ethically define what is happening in this situation?
2. If you had kept the morphine turned on, would you be letting him die or causing him to die? Is there a difference? How do you justify your actions?
3. What is at stake in this situation?

Notes

1. Matter of *Quinlan*, 70 NJ 10(1976), 355 A2d 647 (NJ1976).
2. *Omnibus Budget Reconciliation Act of 1990*, Pub L No. 101–508 ** 4206, 4751.
3. Suicide Act 1961 c 609-and10 Eliz-2 (on line).

References

Brown, N. K., Thompson, D. J., Bulger, R. J., & Laws, E. H. (1971). How do nurses feel about euthanasia and abortion? *American Journal of Nursing, 71*(7), 1413–1416.

Butts, J., & Rich, K. (2005). *Nursing ethics across the curriculum and into practice*. Boston: Jones and Bartlett.

California Natural Death Act (1976). Encyclopedia of Death and Dying (on line).

Carroll, P. R. (1978). Who speaks for incompetent patients? The case of Joseph Saikewicz. *Trustee, 31*(12), 19, 21–22, 24; www.pubmed.gov.

Catlin, A. J. (2006). Moving a vision forward: Neonatal Palliative Care. In D. J. Mason, J. K. Leavitt, & M. W. Chafee (Eds.), *Politics and policy in nursing and healthcare*. Wahoo, NE: Saunders.

Cohen-Almagor, R. (2004). *Euthanasia in the Netherlands: The policy and practice of Mercy Killing*. Warren, WI: Springer.

Diesser, R. (2005). Schiavo's legacy: The need for objective standards. *Hastings Center Report, 35*(3), 20–22.

Ferrell, B. R., & Covie, N. (Eds.). (2005). *Textbook of palliative nursing*. New York: Oxford University Press.

Ferrell, B. R., & Covie, N. (2008). *The nature of suffering and the goals of nursing*. New York: Oxford University Press.

Kant, I. (1976). Duties towards the body in regard to life. In S. Gorovitz et al. (Eds.), *Moral problems in medicine* (pp. 376–377). Englewood Cliffs, NJ: Prentice-Hall.

Mansson, H. H. (1972). Justifying the final solution. *Omega, 3*, 79–87.

Matzo, M. L. (2006). *Palliative care nursing: Quality of care to the end of life*. Warren, WI: Springer.

McIntyre, A. (2004). Doctrine of Double Effect. *Stanford Encyclopedia of Philosophy* (on line).

National Association of Neonatal Nurses (2006). Position Statement #3015: NICU Nurse Involvement in Ethical Decisions. (on line – NANN-Publications).

President's Commission for the Study of Ethical Problems in Medicine and Biomedical and Behavioral Research: *Deciding to Forgo Life-Sustaining Treatment* (1983). Washington, DC: United States Government Printing Office.

Resolve Through Sharing (RTS) Position paper on Perinatal Palliative Care. La Cross, WI: Gundersen Luthern Medical Foundation, 2008 (numerous online sites).

Saver, C. (2008). Central Florida clinicians handle organ donation after cardiac death. http://include.nurse.com. Nurse.com.

Taylor, C. (1995). Medical futility and nursing. *Image: Journal of Nursing Scholarship, 27*(4), 301–306.

Tolstoy, L. (1967). The death of Ivan Ilych. *Great short works of Leo Tolstoy* (pp. 245–302). New York: Harper Row.

CHAPTER 9

Mental Illness and Developmental Disability

INTRODUCTION

This chapter has two foci: (a) mental illness and (b) developmental disability. Generally speaking, people who possess these attributes share some similar ethical problems but they also have some differences between them. Ethical issues for people with mental illness will be discussed first.

The long history of social evolution has engaged the human species in an endless struggle to understand, predict, influence, and control human behavior. The notion of the common good is invoked in most instances to justify coercing an individual to conform to social mores. Historically, the tyranny of the majority has had limited results, especially in private life, since the machinery of repression has had no efficient ways to cope with the deviance and nonconformity in the confines of an individual's own home and in private relationships. Laws developed in this area of life functioned mostly as expressions of public morality rather than as incursions on private liberty. However, more recently developed control methods have now made it possible to exact conformity with greater reliability and less potential for resistance. Increasingly, we have the technology to effectively engineer consent and eliminate personal license but still leave individuals with the feeling that they are free. This may appeal as a therapeutic tool to those who work with the "hard-core" criminal or the severely mentally ill; however, behavior control developments, used widely, can also serve to unhinge the conventional political morality essential to modern democracy. The basic ethical problem in behavior control is how to maintain personal liberty in situations where suppression of liberty can be rationalized, not only by the needs of the common welfare, but also by the individual's well-being.

The potential success of behavior control techniques to change people—prison inmates, substance abusers, mentally ill patients, people seeking psychiatric help for self-fulfillment and self-realization, the developmentally disabled, and people with dementia—has become a source of controversy within the larger debate as to society's proper response to deviant behavior. Unintended consequences mean that reforms and innovations often have effects that are social in nature contrary to the stated purpose of the intended goals and become a central concern in developing techniques to control behavior. The original intent of asylums for the mentally ill was to provide protective settings with treatment and humane conditions, but over time this approach also had the unintentional consequence of turning asylums into warehouses for mentally ill persons, where loss of individuality, depersonalization, and dehumanization resulted (Porter, 2003). The concerns surrounding behavior control and its unintended consequences can be understood in the context of three social dilemmas that mental hospitals share with other institutions of social control:

1. How does the institutional social structure affect attempts at treatment and rehabilitation or protective care?
2. How can these institutions meet both the demands of society and the needs of the individuals they serve?
3. What kind of oversight should there be in the development and application of behavior control techniques?

During the 1950s and 1960s, policy makers recognized that prisons and mental hospitals fell far short of meeting the goals set by society. Critics, both in and out of the mental health field, traced this failure to a number of variables, including the basic one that the social structure of these institutions did not always support their stated goals and could undermine their purpose. The recognition of these problems led to three changes that affected the "total institution" nature of the mental hospital (Goffman, 1961). First, to alter the mental hospital social structure, the therapeutic community concept became a major reform movement. Second, the community mental health movement began to curb the negative aspects of maintaining a patient in the same institution over a long period of time. This change resulted in a shift from almost total reliance on public institutions with their involuntary incarceration and treatment to a more voluntary and pluralistic system known as deinstitutionalization. An awareness of and concern for the civil rights of the involuntarily committed mentally ill during the 1960s was one aspect of a broader social consciousness concerning the rights of women and ethnic minority groups as full participants in American life. Economics, however, also played a role in deinstitutionalization because housing patients in large institutions was expensive. The third change was the development of more sophisticated, more effective, and more efficient behavior control technologies. While the history of behavioral control technology includes electroshock therapy, psychosurgery, behavior modification, and other psychological techniques, it is psychotropic drugs that have had the most influence in shifting the place of care from large institutions to the community.

The issue of behavioral control, however, did not end with the move to a community locus of care. Homelessness is one area where the issue of behavioral control can be seen. Community care done well, like institutional care done well, is expensive, and inadequate funding and housing lead to increasing numbers of the homeless mentally ill (Breakey & Thompson, 1998). The 1980s deinstitutionalization occurred at a time of decreases in the tax base for public services, and the consequent poor services provided were excused because the government could not do anything more. These sentiments continue to the present and result in persistent and seriously inadequate funding for mental health services. Also during the past

30 years, private insurers have dramatically limited mental health coverage for policy holders. As mental health services decreased and state mental hospitals closed, the mentally ill became visible to society with increasing demands to control this deviancy. In the absence of adequate services, jails have become an option for the seriously mentally ill. This is a return to the Middle Ages. The focus here is on the mental health system, but comments about the prison system are needed. The jail and prison populations have swelled over the past 20 years largely with nonviolent offenders because of the war on drugs. Should this lead us to question the wisdom of the policy? Second, in this era of general resistance to taxes, jail construction and operations have received fairly widespread social endorsement. The mentally ill are either living on the streets or increasingly incarcerated in jails, and the health care providers who work in jails interface with both systems of social control (Norman, Parrish, 2002).

Regardless of setting, behavioral control technology raises basic legal and ethical questions about the rights of patients and the role of staff members who some view as double agents—as regulatory agents for the state and as therapeutic agents for the patient. Does this create a conflict-of-interest problem for staff?

Before proceeding, it will be helpful to define behavior control technology and to consider the fundamental problems of deviancy and coercion. Behavior control technology is getting people to do someone else's bidding and has been depicted in several classic, fictional, and nonfiction accounts (Condon, 1959; Huxley, 1932; Koestler, 1970; Orwell, 1959). In the broadest sense, behavior control can be understood as a special form of behavioral change. In a psychiatric setting, treatment offered to or imposed on a patient may be designed to satisfy the wishes of others. Behavioral change that satisfies others—the community or family—may or may not satisfy the patient's wishes to change. The use of behavior control with the mentally ill has been questioned on the grounds that such treatment deprives patients of the fundamental right to choose their course of action. As behavior control technology develops and becomes more available, and as the psychiatric categories expand to include more attitudes and behaviors defined as deviant, numerous ethical questions arise. Preventive psychiatry continues to define more problems of human behavior within its jurisdiction, yet the critics maintain that its practitioners are unable to cope with its present scope. This inability to deliver the goods may be considered both an ethical problem and a safeguard against unchecked power. With recent research probing the biological base of major mental illnesses, some future ethical questions will differ from those in behavior control today.

DEVIANCY AND MENTAL ILLNESS

Every society has its rules and social norms. It is generally expected in a society that a majority of the people will conform to these rules and norms most of the time. In addition, every society has its nonconformists, for example, artists with a bohemian lifestyle, which most communities will tolerate without attempting to control if such a lifestyle does not deviate too much from the established norm. The nonconformists considered deviant and social problems in our society are not a homogeneous group, and the characteristics that bring them societal attention are not easy to classify. While attitudes are changing to some extent in some places, the most obvious groups considered deviant in our own society fall into the following nonexclusive categories:

- Medical (the mentally ill)
- Intellectual (the developmentally disabled)
- Chronological (those with senile dementia)
- Social (the alcoholic)
- Economic (other drug abusers)
- Sexual (the homosexual)
- Doctrinal nonconformity (the sociopolitical radical)

These groups share two things in common: their behavior is proscribed or controlled by law, and society has sought them out for treatment instead of punishment. Social norms change and influence the definition of what is deviant. For example, homosexuality has been eliminated from the category of psychopathology. Such change shows the fluidity of the boundaries between normal and abnormal behavior.

Social groups create deviance when they make rules whose infraction constitutes deviance and when they apply those rules to particular individuals and label them as outsiders. Deviance is not solely a quality of the act the person commits, but rather a consequence of the application by others of rules and sanctions on a perceived offender. The deviant person is one to whom that label has successfully been applied, and deviant behavior is behavior that these people engage in.

Those persons we call mentally ill tend to be at variance with the mores and conventions of society. The fact that this condition usually has behavioral rather than physiological symptoms casts those so labeled into the role of the social deviant. Mental illness is not easy to define or to determine, and this becomes compounded because different societies have different tolerance levels for the sort of deviation that becomes labeled as mental illness.

The concept *dangerousness* is the paramount consideration in the legal commitment procedure within our mental health system. However, this was not always the case, and prior to the 1960s, the major consideration was the idea *in need of treatment*. Although some states allow involuntary commitments on the grounds of being *gravely disabled*, which means the inability to find food and shelter, the risk of dangerousness remains the standard in contemporary mental health law. This means that for the mentally ill who are deviant, the justification for civil commitment is a provable likelihood of dangerous acts toward the self or others. Despite the fact that the mental health field does not possess the tools to determine, with precision, those who will be dangerous, the prediction of dangerousness remains a key factor. Three explanations are possible. First, the courts continue to demand that mental health providers make these assessments. Second, the practical concern that the mentally ill who are violent increasingly comprise the inpatient population—a result of the overall decrease in beds combined with the restriction of admission to that of danger to self or others. Finally, the mentally ill can no longer be committed for indeterminate lengths of stay. This means that commitment is no longer a single solution, with the result that the management of the dangerous mentally ill in the community, difficult in its own right, creates anxiety for the community. Dangerousness, like some other things, is, to some extent, in the eye of the beholder. The concept of dangerousness can be viewed as a social construction in that nursing personnel on locked inpatient psychiatric units can define patients as dangerous even when the patient has not done anything that is dangerous to self or others. While the general public tends to associate dangerousness with mental illness, numerous experts have pointed to the inadequacy of the criteria for predicting who will commit a dangerous act. Although the vast majority of the seriously mentally ill are no more dangerous than the general population, there is a subset that are. Among this subset, substance abuse, noncompliance with medication, and a history of violent behavior are important predictors.

Some critiques of the idea that violence can be predicted emphasize that violent behavior is not only a function of personality but also a function of social context. The theory of social context provides one explanation as to why the traditional psychiatric approach, which emphasizes personality, would have limited predictive value. These comments are not intended to imply that no traditional psychiatric clues are valid, only that such validity has yet to be established. The difficulty involved in predicting dangerousness increases when the patient has never actually performed an assaultive act. This problem becomes particularly relevant in involuntary hospitalization situations. The concern is that mental health professionals, since they have no reliable criteria, over predict dangerousness. In such instances, the argument goes that these professionals have stereotyped ideas of the personality attributes of dangerous individuals that have no proven relationship to the occurrence of dangerous acts. Rather, they commit themselves to these stereotypes because of theoretical constructs that cause them to attend selectively to certain data. In addition to the problems of identification and prediction of dangerous behavior, some maintain that neither mental hospitals nor prisons are now capable of treating persons labeled dangerous. It must be seen as a bizarre system of criminal justice that confines mostly those who cannot be identified as dangerous and equally bizarre a mental health system that commits mostly those who cannot be treated.

Most research on the management of violent behavior is based on inpatient settings. The knowledge contributed by such work is important, but it is no longer sufficient as the dangerous mentally ill are being discharged to the community from inpatient settings or they are not being admitted in the first place. While some work on the community management of violent behavior has been done, the complexity of the issues warrants more study.

COERCION AND FREEDOM

In the United States, freedom constitutes a dominant value; however, the structure of organized society depends on defined limits of freedom. The legal system supplies the definitions of permissible behavior and establishes the coercive force that society may use to ensure compliance. Therefore, coercion may not necessarily always be a bad thing. The basis of organized societies depends to a great extent on the right of the state to coerce its citizens to conform to behavioral standards codified in law. We must weigh society's right to coerce against an individual's right to freedom. Furthermore, one needs to think through what constitutes a coerced, as distinguished from a free, act. Freedom, a principle to which psychiatry aspires rather than a concept that it has often employed, has not been incorporated to any extent into a theory of behavior, since psychiatry has difficulty fitting freedom with any theory that tends toward a deterministic view (Gaylin & Jennings, 2003).

Since people's beliefs and experiences form the basis of future behavior, the perception of danger becomes the crucial issue in understanding coercion. If you feel threatened, it is easier to justify coercion on the basis of that perception. To understand coercion, one must understand what threatens individuals and groups. The problem is not so much the coercion involved in physical force and threatening survival itself, but threats to survival equivalents, such as threat of isolation, loss of love, social humiliation, and so on.

As stated earlier, the social order relies to some extent on the state's right to coercion. Along with the legal dimensions of coercion, society has given a moral privilege to coercion when such action is done in the individual's best interest. For example, certain parental behavior coerces children, but society permits this because of the assumption that parents have the child's best interest at heart. Also, in the field of health, coercion has a traditional respectability and legal sanction, and psychiatry, as a branch of medicine, has engaged in coercion. One could say that, in the recent past, the abrogation of the legal rights of the mentally ill, the denial of due process, and the confinement beyond the limits the law tolerated for criminals represent gross examples of coercion.

Morally reflective nurses know that they bear an instrumental relationship to institutionalized medicine, which implies that nursing can become the means for goals set by medical knowledge. A reduction of mechanical restraint never became a compelling professional ideal in the United States, and a therapeutic philosophy of control characterizes most health care institutions. Physical restraint and locked seclusion remained a reality in the management of many troublesome patients. Those nurses who recognize the roles they occupy are particularly sensitive to the potential for coercion and loss of patient autonomy. Those attuned to ethical dimensions of psychiatric nursing practice have repeatedly documented that direct-care nurses experience the balancing of patient moral agency against social control as a central moral concern.

Behavior control includes a broad spectrum of activities: psychiatric therapy, political propaganda, commercial advertising, religious and moral education, and rehabilitation of deviant persons. The major categories of behavior control in the mental health field discussed here are psychotherapy, psychosurgery, and psychopharmacology. Practitioners in the field readily accept the fact that patients should be protected from outright coercion, and this belief has been formalized in statutes and regulations. The idea that the patient should also be protected from more subtle pressures is not only more difficult for many mental health professionals to accept, but also makes the problems of such regulation more difficult.

Psychotherapy

Psychotherapy has been developed through three stages during the 20th century in response to the psychosocial motif dominating society at that time. Stage one began with the development of psychoanalysis around the beginning of the 20th century, when Freud and Breuer first published their works and formed the Psychoanalytic Society in 1902. The psychoanalytic approach to treatment uncovered and exposed unconscious, repressed material and this came to be known as the talking cure. The patients, mostly middle-class women, lived in Victorian Vienna, known for its standards of proper behavior and repression of sexuality. Psychoanalysis offered a viable explanation of the human mind and its desires in conflict with a repressive, controlling society. While psychoanalysis is still practiced, it is mostly limited to the affluent, and even its more commonly utilized descendent, psychodynamic psychotherapy, is increasingly rare. One problem identified with all psychotherapeutic approaches requiring long-term therapy has been the lack of evidence to prove their effectiveness for patients since traditional psychodynamic therapies have not produced empirical validation of treatment efficacy. Two problems arise with attempts to research this area: (a) defining what is to be measured, which rests on the larger problem of the definition of *normal* or *healthy* and (b) the methodology, to evaluate possible long-range effects of psychotherapy on both individuals and society. While these are legitimate issues, it is important to note that these criticisms arose within a context of complex social factors that changed the focus of treatment from predominately psychological to predominately biological approaches. This shift is not a novel phenomenon but another phase in the swinging pendulum that has occurred between these two competing systems seeking to explain and control human behavior.

The potential for using psychotherapy as a coercive tool of social control increases in the case of involuntary commitment. Psychotherapy can be based on the social and economic biases of the therapist rather than on the patient's behavior, and then can become a coercive tool operating mainly on those very groups that are least able to change the social context in which their problems arise.

Stage two occurred during the 1950s and 1960s, with the development of psychotherapy based on principles of conditioning. *Behavior modification* became the generic name for those methods emphasizing a behaviorist orientation. Another activist treatment, crisis intervention, led to the establishment of crisis intervention centers where clients could come in or telephone at any time in an attempt to deal with their problems. (The 9-1-1 emergency number was instituted in 1967.) These two approaches shared several things: direct attack on the symptoms presented, without going into the underlying cause; short duration of therapy; and the possibility of a more technological basis for therapy than was available in previous therapeutic approaches. Stage two represents a shift from treating causes to treating symptoms.

Stage three grew out of the affluence and leisure that the large middle class had achieved in the late 1960s and the early 1970s, when society passed from the age of anxiety to the age of ennui. The achievement of values and meaning in life became an overriding preoccupation for many. Psychotherapy shifted away from a focus on the relief of discomfort and pain to meeting the demands of those seeking a richer life with deeper experiences and relationships. As indicated in stage one, the developments in stages two and three, separately or in combination, can also serve as coercive tools of social control. Developments from all three stages continue to function to meet the different needs of individuals with a great variety of reasons for seeking help or having it imposed on them. But psychotherapy has fallen out of social favor. One reason for this is the economics of this care—psychotherapy is expensive in time and money. It is difficult to know exactly how economics figured in the present shift to the primacy of biology with drug treatment but it certainly played a role. In spite of its markedly diminished status, psychotherapy still has its adherents among both practitioners and those who seek it.

In addition to the issues in each stage of the development of psychotherapy, there are other problems, clinical, social, and ethical, that make this form of treatment problematic. Among these are the homeless mentally ill and the large numbers of the young, chronically mentally ill who often have dual diagnoses as a result of their mental illness and drug taking. These populations represent a failure in the social movement of deinstitutionalization, the goal of which was to empty mental hospitals and help the mentally ill enter society.

Substance abuse is an acute social problem, and society has declared war on drugs. The fact that great numbers of people are addicted to drugs of all types and that newborn babies begin life addicted have grave potential consequences for society and certainly raises numerous ethical issues. For example, should these drugs be legalized? Should abusers, apprehended by the police, be forced to enter treatment programs, and who will pay for such programs? Should bus drivers, truck drivers, and others whose jobs may do harm to others if performed under the influence of drugs undergo drug testing in order to retain their jobs? Should pregnant women who are on drugs either have an abortion or be placed in a treatment program? What obligations does society have to these babies, to these mothers? Taken together these problems demonstrate the dynamic interaction among the concepts of democracy, social definitions and issues, behavior control questions, and ethical dilemmas.

Behavior control, as a potential ethical dilemma, varies with the different methods of treatment used. Psychotherapy was widely accepted and practiced by therapists as the major means to deal with psychological disorders. It has been less recognized or discussed as a means of controlling people. Long-term insight therapy can be utilized systematically to influence attitudes and values, if not overt behavior, toward conventional norms of conduct. One could, however, argue that because this therapy method is slow, technologically benign, and limited to a relatively small population, the risks of behavior control are few. As behavior changes occur, patients develop an accompanying increase in awareness, enabling them to monitor their own behavior changes to some extent. To a large degree, clients participating in insight therapy are outside large mental hospitals, so the factors of institutional social structure do not affect their lives.

Stage two of psychotherapy, which uses the concept of conditioning, deserves more attention since these techniques have been rigorously criticized as being repressive and dehumanizing. At times, our fascination with technology leads us to overrate the promise as well as the threat of these new techniques. The type of behavior control known as *behavior therapy* or *behavior modification* is one in which the therapist manipulates the environment and the consequences of a person's behavior to change that behavior. The therapist reinforces desired behavior, whereas the undesired behavior receives an adverse response or no reward.

This type of therapy has had limited success because of the difficulty in retaining changed behavior over time. The major question has to do with possible gains as against possible losses. Considerable evidence that people's behavior can be programmed fairly easily now exists. Behavior modification was greatly influenced by behaviorism developed by B. F. Skinner with its emphasis on environmental control and shaping of behavior (Skinner, 1953). The antibehaviorism viewpoint, developed as a reaction to behavior modification and expressed by Carl Rogers and others contended that while the behaviorist approach acknowledges an individual's susceptibility to manipulation by another, it also ignores the possible deleterious impact of this manipulation on the whole person and, in addition, on the manipulator (Rogers, 1955).

Psychosurgery

Psychosurgery, surgery that alters behavior, has almost disappeared from treatment options since the 1970s, but the continued popularity of such films as *Frances* and *One Flew Over the Cuckoo's Nest* has insured that it stays in the public consciousness. Often, improvements in patients' symptoms occurred following psychosurgery but these were largely attributed to decreases in emotional intensity rather than changes in thinking. The initial promise of a miracle cure gave way to a more honest appraisal. Responses to psychosurgery varied and could be related to numerous factors. For example, one reason was that patients who underwent this surgery developed dementia that could not be attributed to other causes. Other reasons included increased questioning of the procedure by the media; disputes between psychiatrists and neurosurgeons over different techniques of lobotomy; the development of chlorpromazine (Thorazine) in the 1950s; and the growing popularity of psychotherapy and psychoanalysis. By the late 1960s, psychosurgery had been dramatically curtailed but not obliterated, and some surgery continued to be performed until the very early 1970s. The social climate of the 1960s challenged the perceived wisdom of the status quo. The challenge came largely from Vietnam War protestors, civil rights advocates, the Black Panthers, women's rights advocates, alternative health care advocates, flower power, the sexual revolution, and advocates for the elderly such as the Gray Panthers. These social movements signaled a distrust of traditional authorities and their power.

Psychopharmacology

Mass media has informed us about the pharmacological developments potentially enabling control of human emotions and mental functioning as well as the extent of drug use in the United States. Earlier we had thought of psychotropic drugs as limited to use by patients diagnosed as psychotic or depressed. But now relatively normal people increasingly use these agents to cope with the stresses in daily life. The production and distribution of psychotropic drugs are a major component of the drug industry. At one time, diazepam or Valium was the most widely prescribed drug in the country, especially for women; this may have been replaced by Prozac.

Yet, Americans seem to have an ambivalent relationship to drugs and vacillate between acceptance and intolerance of drugs such as opium, cocaine, and marijuana. Presently, ours is a drug culture, and many people think a visit to the doctor is a waste of time unless they receive pills, and the medical professional often reinforces this attitude. We eagerly endorse and demand the latest therapeutic drug for *us* while condemning street drug use by *them*—we declared war on those drugs and appointed a drug czar. The drug subculture has grown to become a major social, economic, and mental health problem. This subculture exists as part of a larger culture in which drugs are readily seen as "magic bullets."

Psychotropic drugs have been divided into three categories, depending on the purpose for which they are used: (a) as therapeutic agents for the treatment of psychiatric disorders, (b) for nontherapeutic purposes, such as recreation or personal enjoyment, and (c) to enhance performance and capabilities. Of the techniques developed that can be used for controlling behavior, drugs are among the most widely disseminated and readily available. In each of these categories, ethical issues arise, including that of coercion, which can be a special problem in category one. There are numerous reasons why mentally ill persons or those with behavioral problems may not want to take psychotropic medications. Some people may not see themselves as having a problem in need of control. Some medications interfere with the performance of specific skills or abilities. Several of these drugs have numerous, severe side effects. Health care providers sometimes fail to listen to patients as they try to explain their concerns regarding medication. With emphasis on biological therapeutics for mental illness, we forget that even if research were to find the "magic bullet," the patient would have to agree to take it—unless, of course, we are to have a truly totalitarian state. Currently, there is more discussion focused on the rights of the mentally ill to refuse medication and some state laws ensure those rights.

ETHICAL DILEMMAS AND MENTAL ILLNESS

The right to receive treatment and the right to refuse treatment in general, and the right to consent to or decline behavior modification techniques in particular, raise ethical questions. Do therapists satisfy their own interests or those of the patients or some combination of the two? In some situations, the therapist serves a third party, as an employee of an institution whose interests do not necessarily coincide with the interests of the patient. Third parties often apply subtle and sometimes not so subtle pressures that therapists may not be fully aware of or understand. Conflict of interest represents one facet of the wider problem of what values, especially what conflicting values, are served by the mental health field. A major obstacle to a greater awareness of these possible value conflicts is that mental health professionals can assume that they function from a value-free frame of reference. Keenly aware of the patient's conflicts, they may be less inclined to see the conflicts in their own social role. The fact remains that regardless of therapeutic orientation, these professionals can be a party to such conflict.

The larger ethical question in behavior control is the value of personal integrity. The essential question is, does the individual have an inviolable, defensible, absolute right to be himself or herself, whatever or whoever he or she is, the product of whatever heredity and environment is his or her lot, even if deviant or dangerous to self or others? Questions for consideration in discussing behavior control include the following:

- If the individual is a danger to self, does society have the right to intervene to stop him or her from hurting or destroying himself or herself?
- Does society have the right or obligation to protect its members from themselves or from others?
- On what moral ground can the limit be determined where individual rights become outweighed by societal rights?
- Who will decide who is dangerous using what standard?
- How is normalcy to be defined for therapy?
- If a socially deviant person receives psychiatric treatment, should the aim of that treatment be adjustment or adaptation?
- Are there ethical grounds for rejecting some or all of the more potent behavior control techniques, even if they prove to be quite effective?
- When are possible risks from such procedures justified?
- How is informed consent obtained and from whom?
- Is experimentation justified outside of the context of a reasonable belief that the procedure will be therapeutic for the individual?

- If therapists use these techniques increasingly, should there be some type of regulatory mechanism over and beyond informed consent?
- Should such treatment as long-term use of psychotropic drugs or psychosurgery be considered for children?
- If so, which children will be eligible for this treatment, who will decide, and on what grounds?
- Is it ethical to deny such treatment to adults or children, if all other treatment approaches have failed?
- Should brain surgery be used to control violent behavior, even if such behavior is of unknown cause?
- How do behavior control techniques affect the relationship between the patient and doctor, nurse, or family?
- How does the technology affect the distribution of monetary and other resources for medical care?
- Who pays for such treatment?
- What are the possible potential societal implications of behavior control?

Essentially, the basic ethical questions are the following: What kind of behavior should be controlled? Whose behavior is controlled? Who controls? Who decides who controls? How does behavior control affect dignity and freedom? What are the costs of gaining self-control? What social interests justify social control? What instruments of control are warranted to serve the interest of society? These questions highlight the dilemma of maintaining personal integrity versus society's obligation to protect its members. The dilemma of immunity versus forfeiture of rights raises the question of what rights to privacy and inviolability of body and mind a person should lose once he or she has been diagnosed as mentally ill, especially if he or she is committed to an institution. The dilemma of procedural rights is concerned with what rights a patient has to the procedural protection from the suspension, waiver, or forfeiture of these basic rights. The dilemma of rights and goods concerns the possible conflict between the person's right to be different and her or his potential desire to be free from any misery that his deviance causes. The dilemma of informed voluntary consent raises the issues of mental status and legal status as inhibitions to obtaining informed consent. The dilemma of paternalism and authoritarianism raises the questions that John Stuart Mill addressed: What are the limits on the use of coercion, on the kinds of coercion, and on the actions coercively prevented or elicited that one person may use on another in the name of the latter's own good (Mill, 1978)? The fact that those using intervention techniques may be doing so with therapeutic intent does not alter either the paternalistic or the authoritarian character of such use under certain circumstances. The dilemma of deceptive labeling concerns the issue of when enforced treatment, especially that involving irreversible effects, becomes primitive control under a false therapeutic label. In 1971, Kittrie developed a *Therapeutic Bill of Rights* articulating ethical views relevant to behavior control today. It outlines individual rights of people who are mentally ill and balances these rights with notions of the common good (Kittrie, 1971).

IMPLICATIONS FOR NURSING PRACTICE

The nurse's role in psychiatric settings has ranged from custodial keeper of the keys to skilled therapeutic agent. In any of these roles, nurses have the power to influence and determine, in part, the patient's course of treatment, since they observe and interact with the patient. Nurses in all specialties have such influence, to some extent, but in the mental health field, it takes on special significance because the illness is tied to behavioral symptoms. Mental health nurses, like other staff members, have their own attitudes and value system, which affect their definitions of mental illness and mental health. These attitudes and values become a factor in their encounters with patients. For example, the field of psychiatry has, on paper, changed its concept of homosexuality. Mental health workers in this country are members of the larger society, which in some places has had, and continues to have, deeply ingrained negative attitudes toward homosexuality. These negative attitudes extend to some of society's most marginalized people, such as drug abusers, sex offenders, prostitutes, and criminals. Yet, these people often find themselves in the mental health system and working with them can pose a moral problem for nurses.

Another ingrained cultural attitude is the double standard of mental health for men and women and the differences in the treatment of women in our society.

Declaring women *insane* and incarcerating them was condoned by all states, and in some states, women exercising economic independence was reason enough for being declared insane. For a revealing moral indictment of the treatment of women within the mental health system, an indictment in the words of the women themselves, read *Women of the Asylum* (Geller & Harris, 1994).

Once a person enters the mental health system as a patient, the nurse becomes a major source of information regarding that person's behavior. This is especially so in inpatient settings where longer contacts can occur between nurse and patient and where the nursing staff is the only group to work a 24-hour day. Many decisions regarding treatment occur in team meetings, and the nurse affects the discussion by either providing information or withholding it. What is reported and how it is said influences others' perceptions of the patient. In Rosenhan's classic study, pseudopatients gained admission to mental hospitals by saying they heard voices. Once admitted, they found themselves indelibly labeled with the diagnosis of schizophrenia, in spite of their subsequent normal behavior. They kept field notes for the research project and the nurses charted that these "patients" engaged in "compulsive writing." Only the other patients suspected that these pseudopatients were not mentally ill and were there for other reasons. The staff was unable to acknowledge normal behavior within the hospital milieu. In such a setting, staff members tended to see pathology more than they saw normal behavior (Rosenhan, 1973).

Another potential problem with ethical dimensions that adds to the larger problem of behavior control is whether nurses take the patient seriously. Does the diagnosis of mental illness affect our attitudes toward this category of humans so that we do not take seriously what they say or do? Because someone is "crazy," it may be easier to dismiss him or her by not believing what he or she communicates, since it does not reflect reality. Such an attitude may be supported by the reward system of the institution where the nurse works as an employee.

A paternalistic attitude tends to reduce adult patients to the status of a child and permits the nurse to violate the patient's rights, such as the right to participate in decisions influencing their welfare. Paternalism is interference with a person's liberty of action with the exclusive justification that it is for the welfare, good, happiness, needs, interests, or values of the person being coerced. Some think that self-protection or the prevention of harm to others is a sufficient warrant; however, as stated earlier, the mental health field lacks tools for predicting dangerousness. Others think that the individual's own good is never sufficient warrant for the exercise of compulsion either by the society as a whole or by its individual members. Currently, few theorists are willing to defend the traditional type of paternalism in which health professionals imposed their own values and wills upon patients. Patient autonomy is now thought to be extremely valuable and has been given great moral weight. Of concern is that this claim for autonomy is being used to justify a new form of paternalism.

Nurses in all settings can interfere with a patient's liberty of action. Mental health nurses are in a particularly good position to do so, since either the patient has sought help with his or her behavioral problems or the patient has been committed by legal procedures. In the former case, the staff may feel they have been given license to make decisions for the patient's own good, in the latter, the staff may think they have both the right and obligation to interfere with the patient's liberty of action.

These ideas, influencing decisions regarding mental status and treatment, not taking the patient seriously, and paternalism, can play a part in discussions of using behavior control techniques. Nurses participate in individual and group psychotherapy and in behavior modification programs and have influence on decisions about drugs, such as type, dosage, and frequency. Drugs make the patient more amenable to other types of therapy, such as psychotherapy and also make the patient more manageable from a nursing point of view. This raises some ethical issues around the problem of the double-agent role in which the nurse must follow institutional norms and rules while meeting the patient's needs. The nurse is an agent both for the institution and for the patient. This can cause a conflict for the nurse. To the extent that nurses are aware of these issues, they can examine them not only from a clinical perspective but also from an ethical one (Abma & Widdershoven, 2006).

At times the mental health field can promise more than it can deliver given the knowledge and technology it has available. This raises ethical problems and dilemmas. The technology available has potential for abuse with regard to behavior control. The single most important factor in the intelligent use of such techniques is ethically grounded clinicians who, for moral reasons, hesitate and think through the clinical and ethical implications of their actions. This cannot be overstated. We live in a violent society, and we can be impelled to exercise violence even as we attempt the understandable and laudable goal of controlling it.

DEVELOPMENTAL DISABILITY

Any discussion of ethical dilemmas and the developmentally disabled must take into account the concept of respect for persons. Private morality concerns itself with respecting the distinctive human endowment in ourselves, whereas public morality is concerned with respecting the distinctive human endowment in others. Private morality and public morality represent two aspects of a single, fundamental moral principle. We feel brotherly or sisterly love, *agape*, and respect toward those regarded as persons. This notion leaves open to debate as to who or what properly and truly constitutes a person we respect.

The concept of *person* has a long and complex history within philosophy. Importantly, persons came to be seen as beings in themselves and not merely instrumental to the ends of others. This meaning became particularly important to Immanuel

Kant, a supreme representative of the Age of Enlightenment, who argued that the distinctive endowment of a human being is the ability to reason. For Kant, the possession of a rational will is the quality that gives a human being absolute worth because it is through willingness to do one's duty that one becomes a member of the moral universe. In this way, the word *person* comes to mean more than a certain kind of being, in this case a human being, as contrasted with another kind of being, for example, a cat or a bird. Rather, for Kant, the term *person* conveyed a certain moral status, and for that reason, a person cannot be used as a means to another's end (Kant, 1948). Throughout the history of Western thought, the ability to reason has been associated with language and the capacity to manipulate symbols. Kant's thesis has profoundly influenced directly or indirectly our attitudes toward a number of groups, including the developmentally disabled.

The concept of a *person* is an evaluative concept with the force of "that which makes a human being valuable" implied in it. But the questions remain: Why do we respect or value a person? What makes a human being a person? In the field of developmental disability, as we move along the continuum from severely to borderline disabled, do we perceive each individual as a person or do we draw the line based on moral reasoning ability and think only of some on the continuum as persons we respect? If personhood is *not* dependent on moral reasoning ability, what is it that indicates that someone is a person and what is it about a person who requires our respect and why?

The term *person* seems to refer to a cluster of features including *biological factors* (descended from humans; having a certain genetic makeup); *psychological factors* (having a concept of self and of one's interests and desires; the ability to use language and other symbols); *rationality factors* (the ability to reason and draw conclusions and the ability to learn from past experiences); *social factors* (the ability to work in groups, the ability to recognize and consider the interests of others, and the abilities to love and sympathize); and *legal factors* (the ability to own property and inherit goods, being subject to the law and protected by it, and citizenship). This is not a list of necessary and sufficient conditions for personhood but simply features that are more or less typical of those who are referred to as "persons."

If individuals lack some of these biological, psychological, and rationality factors, do they fail to qualify as persons? Is respect for them as persons dependent on which factors are present and which are lacking? Or, do individuals merely need to be members of the human community to be counted as persons? Respect for them is then dependent on whether or not the community values them and accords them full rights and responsibilities as members of the community. These questions point to the complexity of the concept. Confusion may result from the fact that the same word, *person*, is used in two senses: as a kind of ontological being and as a being in the moral or evaluative sense, that is, as a being who is held accountable for his or her actions. The term can be so confusing as to advocate for its removal from the discourse of health care ethics, arguing that the work of health care concerns human beings. We have some sympathy with this view and would reframe the issue from a concern over personhood to one of respect for human beings.

Respect can mean several things: esteem for some particular talent or capacity; regard for agency, which refers to the capacity of someone to manage his or her own affairs; a recognition of limitations; and regard for class membership, in this case, the class of human beings. Respect in the sense of regard for agency reflects the issues of autonomy, such as the capacity for voluntary action and the capacity to give reasons for those actions. Many developmentally disabled people can do these things to varying degrees. Yet, when someone is profoundly disabled and cannot do these things, some believe that these individuals are still owed respect because they are human beings. Do you agree or not? Why?

Human beings are a class of beings that have a certain embodiment and the capacity for consciousness and/or social interaction. Therefore, they have rights and responsibilities that may vary according to a variety of factors, and they have a moral claim on other members of the community. We depend on each other for support and protection in ways that make the interests of all human beings of special importance to us. The advantage of the term *human being* circumvents the difficulty associated with the concept of person in philosophy, with its focus on rationality. This is particularly important when discussing those individuals whose capacity for rationality is compromised. Our position is that mentally and physically disabled individuals and persons in a coma are worthy of our respect simply because they are human beings.

The ethical dilemmas with the developmentally disabled include how we define developmentally disabled and the consequences of that definition; problems encountered by the developmentally disabled in institutions and in the community regarding their rights; and the moral reasoning that society uses in balancing its resources and values to determine the risks and benefits for the individual and for society itself. Consider the ethical issues of respect for the autonomy of developmentally disabled people. If we believe that support for the enactment of autonomy is central to the ethical treatment of one another, we must ask what autonomy might mean for developmentally disabled individuals. It is not enough to offer choices, but those choices must be meaningful, because it is through our identification with meaningful choices that we define who we are. Practitioners working with the developmentally disabled using behaviorism might take issue with this notion but they, nonetheless, stress the complexity of the idea of choice and the ethical obligation to avoid coercion. This is particularly important because the act of choosing, which involves an evaluation of consequences, is a difficult task for those with limited verbal or symbolic capacities.

The concern is how society fulfills its duties and obligations to safeguard the basic rights of mentally and physically disabled individuals when they cannot, by virtue of their disabilities, completely do so by themselves. The usual rights of the developmentally disabled to defend include the right to family living, educational opportunities, treatment and habilitation services, employment, support in the development of contracts, and confidentiality in personal records. Their special rights include qualified advocacy and guardianship capacity; protection against use of drugs and behavior modification techniques including experimental procedures; counseling and safeguards regarding reproduction; and intelligent exposure to life situations involving risk (Gostin, 2007).

DEFINITION AND LABELING

Some people, including some health care providers, speak of developmental disability as if it referred to a single capacity, most commonly constructed as IQ, or intelligence quotient, rather than a range of abilities across a variety of domains. However, this disability is a state of impairment rather than a single entity and can have multiple causes. Yet, precisely because it is fluid, the definition of developmental disability has been fraught with difficulties and is frequently unsatisfactory. Contemporary ideas of developmental disability are associated with IQ, with its origins in the 1800s. The following scale is often used: borderline, 68–85; mild, 52–67; moderate, 36–51; severe 20–35; and profound under 20. Mental disability, ultimately a social attribute, comprises at least three components: organic, functional, and social. The organic component we refer to as impairment, the functional component as disability, and the social component as handicap.

DEVELOPMENTAL DISABILITY: LAW, ETHICS, AND SOCIAL POLICY

While law and ethics are not the same, they stand in important relationship to each other. Laws have significant ethical implications because they structure a society, thereby setting up minimal standards of expectation. Rights, when codified legally, incur binding obligations. The relationship between the law and issues of developmental disability is complex and fluid, reflecting many social factors and influencing public policy. For example, as a result of the work of the Kennedy family, social consciousness was awakened, concrete services improved, and legal rights procured; in short, social policy was altered. Social policy is a form of collective action, and for developmental disability, four perspectives have been identified: protecting society; protecting the disabled individual; helping society to accommodate the individual; and assisting the individual to participate fully in social life. The next discussion illustrates the intersection of law, ethics, and public policy. These are sterilization, confinement, and the Americans with Disabilities Act.

Although sterilization is no longer a widespread practice for the mentally ill and mentally disabled, its lessons are instructive for many reasons. Most importantly, it shows how specific procedures can become enactments of ideas whose purpose is to justify excluding others from participation in the goods of social life. On the face of it, sterilization might readily be seen as the solution to a legitimate concern for the well-being of children born to certain people. But too often, such solutions are unreflective and morally suspect. There are at least three ethical problems with sterilization.

The first is the relation between sterilization and eugenics, a social movement in the United States of America during the 20th century aimed at maintaining a genetically pure race by prohibiting interracial marriage and engaging in the sterilization of the mentally handicapped. Second, the focus on sterilization can obscure the question of what good parenting involves and who is capable of enacting it. Third, sterilization of developmentally disabled citizens is a power-sanctioned procedure by which the state, in conjunction with medical authority, dictates what kind of life is possible for these individuals. Such decisions can too easily be made without understanding the perspectives of those who will be affected and failing to do so is a moral wrong. In a representative democracy, we, as individuals, bear a great deal of responsibility for the policies of our government because we vote for people who will take action in one way or another. To put it differently, the state is not just *them*—it is *us*.

Another issue that illustrates the intersection of law, ethics, and social policy is confinement. In some states, it is legally easier to involuntarily commit a developmentally disabled person to a hospital than a mentally ill person. The rationale for such difference is the claim that it is easier to diagnose developmental disability than mental illness, greater accuracy in predicting dangerous behavior among the develop-mentally disabled, and less invasive treatment for them.

Values are embedded in all of our social practices, including the laws and social policies we adopt. What are the values underlying the Americans with Disabilities Act (ADA) and how are they enacted in day-to-day life for the disabled individuals and the worlds of which they are a part? While the general values in this act are fairness, equality of opportunity, and beneficence, there are significant ambiguities that arise because these values can conflict. For example, equality of opportunity can be understood in two ways. The first says that standards used to evaluate someone must apply equally to everyone, independent of race, religion, gender, age, poverty, and physical or mental disability. These factors cannot be used against anyone but neither can they be used to help. A second view holds that precisely because some people are more disadvantaged than others, it is unfair to treat everyone in the same way. These two perspectives illustrate the tension in the relationship between the individual and the group, and when the individual is disabled, conflicts in values can be heightened. The example of the child who can attend a regular school but requires an educational aide in constant attendance illustrates this point. If the school board provides this service, will cuts need to be made elsewhere, cuts that might include services to all children? The way we define equal opportunity has critical implications for the allocation of resources. The main moral and social question raised by the application of the ADA is this: Should we remain committed to the rights and welfare of those with severe disabilities while placing limits on their claims? The answer to this question will continue to unfold as the ambiguities come to light and society makes choices (Liao, Savutescu, & Sheehan, 2007).

ETHICAL IMPLICATIONS FOR NURSING PRACTICE

An encounter with developmentally disabled persons can be experienced as a challenge to the most fundamental core of our own personhood. We may react to this as an affront with a variety of feelings, including thankfulness that we are as we are and guilt that we live in a world of "haves" and "have-nots." This latter world is not simply one of physical and cognitive intactness; it is also a political, social, and, above all, economic world. We have lived in a society that tends to espouse economic individualism where a significant portion of people believed that government cannot or should not be about helping people. Perhaps another aspect of the emotions that can be experienced with the loss of a perfect child is the fear of providing for the child in a society that is not structured to include the less than perfect. Political change with a philosophy more focused on the common good can lessen these larger ethical problems but will not eliminate them because of finite resource to be allocated. This is the ethical issue of distributive justice.

In attempting to cope with such an encounter, any feelings of repulsion and disgust can not only prevent us from examining the roots of our reaction but also have wide-ranging effects on our definition of the situation and on how to deal with the moral claims that the developmentally disabled have on us as individuals, as nurses, and as citizens. Our attitudes also will determine how we think the resources of society should be allocated and how much, and what we think the developmentally disabled should receive. The concept of *distributive justice* provides us with a moral framework within which to make these decisions.

Obviously, nurses must first sort out their own feelings about and attitudes toward the developmentally disabled. Such a sorting out will need to take into account the concept of human being and where one draws the line, if at all, with regard to the extent of the disability and the consequences of such action. The following are some of the questions raised:

- What attitudes do I have toward the developmentally disabled?
- What attitudes should I have, and why?
- Do I tend to stereotype all the developmentally disabled and view them as a category rather than as individuals with differences?
- What moral principles have I used to think through my ethical position vis-à-vis the disabled?
- What moral claims do the disabled have on me as a professional?
- What moral claims do the disabled have on society? How do we articulate these claims within the concept of distributive justice?

As the field of genetics further advances, nurses—clinicians, educators, and researchers, individually and collectively—along with other health professionals and concerned citizens must become more knowledgeable about the implications of this research. Decisions and research findings in this field affect all of us now as well as future generations. The need to weigh the potential risks and possible benefits on the future course of human evolution is not of mere academic interest. Our deep-rooted concepts of ourselves and our relationship to the universe may need to be reappraised in this process. This has enormous consequences, not only for the developmentally disabled but for all of us. Value judgments inevitably have played, and will continue to play, an important part in determining the direction society takes on this scientific and ethical issue. One can only wonder if the insights and humility gained from encounters with the developmentally disabled will help in this task before us. As the largest segment of the health industry, nurses have some valuable input for this debate. In all of these ethical dilemmas, the moral virtue of compassion and the moral principles of justice and utility, or the greatest possible balance of good over evil, have a part in our concept of obligations to the developmentally disabled, as well as to the rest of us, now and in the future (Odom, Horner, Snell, & Blacher, 2007).

CASE STUDY I   Mentally Ill

Mary Elizabeth is from a large and well-to-do family. She is 24 years old and living on the streets. Her family has paid to have her admitted to many expensive private psychiatric facilities for treatment of her schizophrenia. Mary Elizabeth always signs herself out. Since she is not judged to be dangerous, she cannot be held against her will.

Her symptoms can be well controlled with psychotropic medication. However, she does not take the drugs and says she does not like the way she feels when she is on them. She writes beautiful poetry and says she finds "my own reality" much more interesting than the boring and tedious life she experiences when on the medication. She prefers the friends she makes on the street to the dullness of "so-called normal people."

Her sister arranges to have her poetry published and sends the meager proceeds to Mary Elizabeth. She is occasionally picked up for vagrancy, however, and brought in for treatment. Her parents are always contacted. Mary Elizabeth does not maintain contact with them otherwise.

Suggested Questions for Discussion

1. Does Mary Elizabeth have the right to live in her "own reality"? What are society's rights and responsibilities toward "vulnerable" individuals like Mary Elizabeth?
2. Should Mary Elizabeth be coerced to take her medications? How? Why? By whom?
3. What responsibility do Mary Elizabeth's parents have for her?

CASE STUDY II   Developmentally Disabled

Sheila is a 30-year-old woman living independently. She works in a workshop making hand-crafted gifts. She was born with congenital heart and lung abnormalities that are progressively worsening. She was recently referred to a transplant center to be evaluated for a possible heart–lung transplant.

The referral center rejected her as a candidate saying that she would not be able to adequately manage her post-transplant care because of her developmental disability. Sheila has Down's syndrome but is highly functional. She appealed to a second center that accepted her. She received the transplant and is now doing very well.

Suggested Questions for Discussion

1. What is the responsibility of the transplant center in seeing that such a scarce resource as organs for transplantation are distributed fairly and equitably? Should such things as cognitive function, self-care capability, and potential for social contribution be considered?
2. Is Sheila less worthy of a transplant than someone with a higher IQ?
3. As a result of Sheila's experience, state legislation barring discrimination in the allocation of organs for transplantation based on preexisting mental or physical disability as defined by the American Disability Act was introduced. How would you respond to this type of legislative initiative?

References

Abma, T. A., & Widdershoven, G. (2006). Moral deliberation in psychiatric nursing. *Nursing Ethics, 13*(5), 546–557.

Breakey, W., & Thompson, J. W. (Eds.). (1998). *Mentally ill and homeless: Special programs for special needs.* Amsterdam: Overseas Publishers Association.

Condon, R. (1959). *The Manchurian candidate.* New York: McGraw-Hill.

Gaylin, W., & Jennings, B. (2003). *Perversion of autonomy.* Washington, DC: Georgetown University Press.

Geller, J. A., & Harris, M. (1994). *Women of the asylum: Voices from behind the walls, 1840–1945*. New York: Anchor Books.

Goffman, E. (1961). *Asylums*. New York: Doubleday.

Gostin, L. O. (2007, July–August). Why should we care about social justice? *Hastings Center Report*, 3.

Huxley, A. (1932). *Brave new world*. New York: Harper & Row.

Kant, I. (1948). *The fundamental principles of metaphysics of morals*. London: Hutchinson's University Library.

Kittrie, N. N. (1971). *The right to be different*. Baltimore: Johns Hopkins University Press.

Koestler, A. (1970). *Darkness at noon*. New York: Bantam.

Liao, S. M., Savutescu, J., & Sheehan, M. (2007, March–April): The Ashley Treatment: Best Interests, Convenience, and Parental Decision-Making. *Hasting Center Report*, 16–20.

Mill, J. S. (1978). *On liberty*. Indianapolis, IN: Hackett Publishing.

Norman, A., & Parrish, A. (2002). *Prison nursing*. Oxford: Blackwell.

Odom, S. L., Horner, R. H., Snell, M. E., & Blacher, J. (2007). *Handbook of developmental disabilities*. New York: Guildford Publications.

Orwell, G. (1959). *1984*. New York: Harcourt, Brace.

Porter, R. (2003). *Madness*. Oxford: Oxford University Press.

Rogers, C. R. (1955). Persons or science: A philosophical question. *Am Psychol, 10*, 267–278.

Rosenhan, D. L. (1973). On being sane in insane places. *Science, 179*(70), 250–258.

Skinner, B. F. (1953). *Walden two*. New York: Macmillan.

CHAPTER 10

Policy, Ethics, and Health Care

Nurses, individually and collectively, are involved in the development and implementation of policy in health care organizations and in the public sector. Policy involvement is supported as an ethical obligation in the current *Code of Ethics for Nurses* (American Nurses Association, 2001). Examples range from policies that determine allocation of nursing care and expertise in hospitals, long-term care facilities, and home care to legislative policies related to advance treatment directives, allocation of resources to and within health care delivery systems, public and private health insurance plans, and research. In this chapter, the term *policy* refers to a course of action or inaction selected from among alternatives in a given context to guide present and future decisions and implementation of those decisions. *ANA's Health Care Agenda* (2005) is an example of a document developed by the nursing profession to influence health policy and health care reform at the federal level (American Nurses Association, 2005). Nursing's history and early leaders such as Florence Nightingale and Lillian Wald illustrate a long tradition of nursing involvement in efforts to influence health policy that affects the public.

Health policy issues involve ethical values that are often not considered explicitly in public debate that usually focuses on economic, legal, and political factors. Yet, ethical values such as fairness in the distribution of the benefits of health care, avoiding harm, and respect for persons should be considered in policy decisions. While more individualistic values, such as professional autonomy, especially for physicians, were emphasized to a great degree during the past three decades, other values such as universal access to health care and more community-oriented values have not been realized. Values of social advocacy as enhancement of the public's health, advocacy for the most vulnerable, and social solidarity as fostering a commitment to community inclusive of different segments of our society are examples of more community-oriented values (Priester, 1992a). Values may be viewed as a set of beliefs and attitudes for which logical reasons can be given. Values influence our perceptions of situations, guide our actions and behavior, are interrelated, and have consequences for individuals and society. Not all values are ethical or moral. Political, economic, and even aesthetic values are other types of values that enter into policy decisions in health care organizations and government sectors.

Debates and decisions about health policy are ultimately based on underlying assumptions about what is valued in society and where health is placed on the list of societal priorities. This reality is significant to nurses as health care providers and to consumers of health care and nursing care, for it means that finite resources are allocated among such competing societal goods as education, housing, defense, and welfare as well as health care. Curative and preventive care, education of health workers, and disease-related research represent competing interests and claims on health dollars.

Fuchs, an economist, pointed out in his now classic book *Who Should Live?* that resources are scarce and have alternative uses and that individuals have different wants and attach different levels of importance to satisfying these wants (Fuchs, 1974). Note that Fuchs talks about wants, not needs. *Needs* can be used as one basis for distribution of benefits and burdens in a just fashion in health policy as in the language of medical necessity used in some health insurance plans to determine health plan benefit packages. The factors mentioned by Fuchs indicate that choices must be made at personal and societal levels in order to resolve issues such as the fairest distribution of resources to health care: who is to choose for communities and nations, how priorities will be set, and how needs and interests of individuals and society will be reconciled in policy development and implementation. These and numerous other challenges reflect value conflicts in our pluralistic society, such as individual freedom of choice in conflict with avoiding harm to others. For example, TB patients who do not comply with medication regimens or patients who have drug-resistant disease put the public at risk. These conflicts are also illustrated in the several goals of health care including containment of costs, delivery of quality health care, and access to health care for all.

Public policy consists of a course of action(s) chosen by government (Kalisch & Kalisch, 1982). Principles guiding these choices are or should be the concern of everyone. Two of the overall purposes of government, as found in the Preamble to the U.S. Constitution, are promoting the general welfare and establishing justice. Public policy is developed within this constitutional framework to meet these general goals. According to Strickland, an historian, the policymaking process consists of deciding on goals for the public good and delineating and activating strategies for achieving these goals. This process requires agreement on both means and ends among those who have effective control over resources, such as money, personnel, and facilities (Strickland, 1972). A national health policy per se does not exist in this country when considering four essential policy aspects: clear statement of purpose, working consensus to achieve the purpose, agreement on means and ends, and continuing fiscal support of composite programs (Strickland, 1972, p. 255). Much American medical care is still focused primarily on the cure of disease and the use of increasingly sophisticated high-tech procedures. At the same time, preventive activities are receiving more attention in business and in health care delivery and education as health care costs continue to escalate.

Relatively few people have insurance coverage for preventive, ambulatory, or long-term care, and millions of individuals and families are uninsured or underinsured for medical care and mental health services at any given point in time. Trends to move more population groups into public and private health insurance plans do not automatically alleviate these problems. We also know that medical care does not always equal health care and that it is only one of several factors that affect health status. Other factors include socio-economic circumstances, race, and age. Additionally, environmental factors involving safety of homes, workplaces, and schools plus the quality of air, food supplies, and water must be taken into account in order to realize comprehensive and ethically supportable health and health-related policies. Environmental quality issues loom ever larger in pursuit of health goals in the new millennium.

Even if the United States does not have a national health policy, the federal budget and health legislation for authorizing appropriations for grants and programs reflect implicit values about societal obligations in and to health care. They provide a foundation for policy making as they reflect the priorities placed on health and health care politically and economically in the overall societal picture. They also impact the allocation of resources to medical care and preventive services; to education of health personnel; and to the provision of personal, community, and environmental health services with profound consequences for the lives and well-being of all people. Currently, resources for health care services are declining even as needs for health and health-related care are increasing. Consider ongoing needs of AIDS patients, people suffering from violence and drug-related trauma, returning injured military, undocumented persons, the chronically mentally ill, and increasing numbers of individuals over 85 as a few examples in our country.

HISTORICAL, LEGISLATIVE, AND POLITICAL BACKGROUND

Selected historical and legislative aspects discussed here demonstrate the ways that values and value conflicts related to health have been part of our history as a country from its early beginnings. Health care has become an increasingly prominent concern on the national policy agenda as costs have ballooned and various interventions, voluntary and mandated, have been used unsuccessfully in attempts to contain these costs over past decades. The increasing numbers of vulnerable people who are uninsured or underinsured and lack adequate access to health care have also focused public concern on health and health care. Government's commitment to health care on the public policy agenda has changed over time and can be traced historically in legislation and appropriations to implement the legislation. These commitments have affected nursing education, nursing research, and the delivery of nursing care directly and indirectly in the past and continue to do so in present times.

Hints of a national health policy can be identified from the time of establishment of the Colonies. Early health measures passed by the Colonies in the 17th century had to do with quarantine for control of communicable diseases such as yellow fever. In the late 18th and early 19th centuries, debate focused primarily on state versus federal authority rather than on health matters per se. Still, Congress went further even then in committing the federal government to more involvement with preservation of citizen health: a vaccination law was passed to make effective cowpox vaccine available to anyone requesting it free of charge. This law was repealed after the wrong vaccine was sent to North Carolina with disastrous results. But a precedent was set for federal involvement in the health of individual citizens (Chapman & Talmadge, 1971).

In the late 1800s, the American Medical Association (AMA) made a distinction between public health and private, individual health. "State medicine" was to benefit communities by dealing with communicable diseases such as smallpox, which could only be controlled through public efforts. Even at that time in our history, there were problems in this public-or-private distinction that rapidly became blurred. Conflicts began to develop between private groups, such as the AMA, and the government over governmental involvement in health. A yellow fever epidemic in the 1870s influenced the authorization of a federal National Board. The Board's duties were rather vague, but in the four years of its existence, it authorized funds for biomedical research (Chapman & Talmadge, 1971, p. 35).

Problems continued with the quarantine law and the authority to enforce it. Eventually, authority was given to the Marine Hospital Service, which became the U.S. Public Health Service in 1912. The Public Health Service was also authorized to do epidemiological research in order to control and prevent the disease. Preventive medicine and the health of the public were still the philosophical bases for government involvement in health matters. Curative medicine and the health of individuals continued to be primarily private concerns (Chapman & Talmadge, 1971, pp. 35–36).

European social and health insurance schemes began to receive attention in the United States in the early 1900s. The climate of economic reform, demands for better working conditions, emergence of labor unions, and passage of the National Health Insurance Act in Britain (1911) stimulated this interest. In the United States, the American Section of the International Association for Labor Legislation promoted the health insurance cause by calling for insurance against accidents, sickness, old age, and unemployment, further indication that health concerns require personal *and* collective action. Government recognition of social and health needs was also reflected in presidential messages, beginning early in the 20th century. Federally sponsored health insurance was mentioned in many of the presidential messages but was not supported with legislation. Interestingly, the AMA was *not* opposed to some form of federal health insurance early in the 1900s (Chapman & Talmadge, 1971, pp. 40–42). This lack of opposition soon ended, and AMA opposition continues to this day with the latest failure of national health reform during the Clinton administration in the early 1990s.

The Great Depression of the 1930s and passage of the Social Security Act in 1935 saw further federal concern over health, even though the Social Security Board had no charge directly related to health insurance when the Act was passed in its final form. In the early 1940s, there were several attempts to pass a bill that would have created a system of federal compulsory health insurance and federal support of medical education. This proposal was strongly opposed by the AMA and never came to a vote. In 1946, the AMA did support the Hill–Burton Bill that provided grants-in-aid through the states for hospital construction. This program was extended in the form of grants for research projects on hospital utilization, construction of nursing homes and other facilities, and hospital modernization projects (Stevens, 1971). This program was part of an overall effort to improve services to citizens and demonstrated the focus on "sick care" in public policy making, rather than on broader health care and prevention.

Legislative forerunners to Medicare and Medicaid appeared in the late 1950s and early 1960s that provided hospital and medical care for the elderly through Social Security and federal aid to the states for the "medically indigent" elderly (Wilson & Neuhauser, 1982). In the 1960s, Medicare (an entitlement program) and Medicaid (a medical assistance program administered by the states) were passed with no provisions for change in the actual structure of health care delivery. Under Medicaid provisions, matching federal grants are made available to the states for medical assistance to groups such as recipients of federally aided public assistance, recipients of supplemental security income benefits, the medically indigent in comparable groups (families with dependent children, the aged, the blind, and the disabled), and other indigent children (Wilson & Neuhauser, 1982, pp. 172–179). Legislative struggles to provide funding for services to medically indigent children and other population groups continue in the new millennium.

Federal Comprehensive Health Planning Amendments were legislated in the late 1960s to encourage state- and area-wide health planning that included providers and consumers. These amendments still did not attempt to change the delivery of health care in any major way. The Health Maintenance Organization Act of 1973 provided financial assistance for development of health maintenance organizations, which include prepaid group medical practice. This is the first deliberate legislative effort at the federal level to reorganize the delivery of health care (Wilson & Neuhauser, 1982, pp. 208–210).

The 1972 Social Security Amendments made major changes in the Social Security Act to include Medicare and Medicaid. One provision in Medicare was for reimbursement of hemodialysis and renal transplantation costs for qualifying individuals who cannot pay their own medical expenses. These amendments also established Performance Standards Review Organizations (PSROs) directed to problems of cost control, quality, and medical necessity of services. In addition, PSROs reviewed professional activities of physicians and other providers (Wilson & Neuhauser, 1982, pp. 176–180).

Establishment of the National Institutes of Health and appropriation of increasing amounts of funding for medical research in the past few decades represent a significant level of governmental support for research to control, cure, and prevent disease. At the same time, Medicaid and Medicare are under increasing attack as containment of health care costs continues to be a major societal concern after failure of the Clinton administration health reform efforts in the early 1990s.

This bird's-eye view of governmental legislative activities related to health reflects value judgments and critical choices made over the years in allocation of finite societal resources, from control of communicable disease to development of medical research and health manpower, financing mechanisms for medical and health care, and efforts to alter health care delivery systems. Federal concerns about the health of citizens are also reflected in other types of legislation not discussed here, such as legislation for regulation of the pharmaceutical industry, health and safety in the workplace, and environmental pollution.

HEALTH CARE POLICY—RECENT DECADES

Radical changes surrounding and influencing health care policy occurred in the past three decades. Rapidly rising health care costs and unsuccessful attempts to deal with them in the context of ever-escalating costs have had a significant role in shaping today's health care system.

Health insurance plans, managed care arrangements, integration of health care facilities into large multi-institutional organizations, outpatient surgeries, urgent care centers, home care, restructuring of the health workforce, implementation of Medicare's Diagnostic Related Groups (DRGs) system, and passage of Medicare Part D for drug payments represent extraordinary changes in financing and delivery of health care in the United States. Most of these efforts demonstrate a policy priority of trying to deal with escalating costs overshadowing other policy objectives (Priester, 1990). This priority and efforts to put it into operation have obscured the impact that these changes have had on ethical values in medicine and health care such as professional autonomy, patient autonomy, advocacy for patients, and the fullest possible access to health care for all (Center for Biomedical Ethics, 1989). Such profound changes in financing and delivery of health care point more clearly than ever to the interface of ethics and politics as society deals with issues such as the allocation and rationing of societal resources in and to health care. They also point to the need for involvement of nurses in organizational and public policy development as nurses are closest to patients and their concerns over time in clinical situations. What are some dimensions of ethically sensitive organizational and governmental health policy?

ETHICAL DIMENSIONS OF HEALTH POLICY

Social scientists Warwick and Kelman, in their now classic writing on the ethics of social intervention in the 1970s, presented four elements for an ethical framework that is still useful for policy development and implementation in the new millennium. Social intervention is regarded by these authors as any planned or unplanned action that changes characteristics of an individual or the pattern of relationships among individuals, often a characteristic of policies in health care organizations and public policy (Warwick & Kelman, 1976). In this discussion, the focus is on changing patterns of relationships as we consider issues in social and political arenas related to health policy and nursing's participation. This framework is also appropriate for identifying and evaluating ethical aspects of existing and developing policies in health care and public health organizations, an issue in the domain of organizational ethics.

Warwick and Kelman discuss four areas of intervention that raise ethical concerns that should be addressed *before* and during policy development and implementation with a goal of more ethically responsible and responsive policy. The four areas of intervention are (Warwick & Kelman, 1976, p. 471):

1. The choice of policy goals that maximize or minimize specific values as in any reimbursement system that has cost containment as a major goal, that is, a goal that maximizes economic values and minimizes human and ethical values such as respect for all persons in need of health care and those who provide that care.
2. The definition of the target of change, that is, who or what is supposed to change—providers, patients and their families, organizations—and identification of how they are involved in the process of policy development, revision, or implementation.
3. Identification of the means and methods chosen to develop and implement policy, ranging from those that are most coercive to those that facilitate what significant stakeholders have chosen to do with provision of the required financial and other types of support and resources needed.
4. Assessment, to the extent possible, of direct and indirect consequences of a proposed policy such as attention to the economic, emotional, social, and psychological costs (a distributive justice concern) to all affected by a proposed policy, such as patients, families, caregivers, and communities.

One example might be a major effort by government to focus policies on preventive health activities in areas of personal and environmental health. Such policy efforts would maximize the value of the greatest good for the greatest number, a more utilitarian or consequentialistic view. At the same time, this might have some negative effects on the values of equity and justice for the mentally ill or the chronically ill elderly. In this example, the choice for targets of change might be individual lifestyles of teenagers and adults and reducing carcinogenic elements in the environment. Methods for inducing change might impinge on values of individual freedom and autonomy or on the freedom of industry to maximize profits. Conflict might occur between groups educating for lifestyle changes, those working for healthier air and water, and those providing care for the acutely ill as they compete for finite societal funding resources. Finally, one has to assess the risks and benefits of various consequences of proposed policy changes on traditional health values such as advocacy for individual patients and the emphasis in managed care arrangements on population-based interventions. If decision makers opt for expenditure of public funds on education for lifestyle changes emphasizing individual responsibility for health, there is the potential for developing a "blame-the-victim" mentality in policy development. What, if any, values such as personal freedom are we willing or unwilling to relinquish or have modified in the interests of a healthier society, containment of health care costs, and preventing harm to the most vulnerable?

A key issue in examining goals for health policy development and the methods chosen for implementing change is the extent to which affected population groups have their values and interests represented in the process—various socioeconomic groups, men, women, children, the employed, the unemployed, the healthy, the sick, providers, and payors. How much control should the affected groups and individuals have in the process of policy development that demonstrates respect for those persons or groups? Whose interests are being served by proposed policy proposals, the providers of preventive health programs, or the populations at risk? Is the power or control of one group of patients or providers strengthened at the expense of another by proposed policies? One example might be the infant population in newborn intensive care and their caregivers in competition for health resources with the frail elderly population and their caregivers. Often, such concerns are not considered because of the difficulty in discerning whose needs and values should take precedence and the difficulty of predicting consequences of particular actions on any selected values, such as respect for individual freedom of choice versus the overall welfare of society (Warwick & Kelman, 1976, p. 476).

Albert Jonsen, a prominent bioethicist, and Lewis Butler, a lawyer and public policy expert, suggest other ways in which ethical concerns might be an explicit aspect of policy debate. In doing so, they also acknowledge challenges that make such dialogue difficult (Jonsen & Butler, 1975). The following are some of those challenges: exploring ethical concerns in policy development often does not provide a ready-made single right decision for action; ethics has its own special language; the common conception that ethics primarily has to do with personal behavior; and policymakers have constituencies with interests and loyalties that ethicists do not.

Yet, both ethicists and policymakers are concerned implicitly or explicitly about what is "good" for an organization or society and for the individuals in either one or both as policy decisions are made. Generally, policymaking situations involve "politics" as making decisions for action that affect power, authority, and status in government, organizations, or even families. Older concepts of politics include the idea that politics is a branch of ethics concerned with ethical relations and duties of governments and other social organizations with a focus on interests of groups rather than on individuals. Politics has also been defined as doing "public ethics." These perspectives negate ethics as *solely* a personal matter or the activities of politicians. Furthermore, politics deals with conflicting needs, interests, and values as do issues in applied ethics.

Jonsen and Butler see "public ethics" as a subset of social ethics, that is, governmental decisions about matters of public concern such as equitable access to benefits of health care and responding to pressing issues such as allocation and rationing of public funds. Three tasks of "public ethics" for public policymakers are (Jonsen & Butler, 1975, pp. 23–24):

1. To articulate the moral principles most relevant to the policy problem under consideration, such as justice, equity, and respect for persons
2. To examine proposed policy choices in view of identified relevant moral principles
3. To rank in order the moral options for particular policy choices

This process is rather like a "moral balance sheet" in terms of which social or economic policies enhance or negate one moral principle and not another, making more explicit the ethical dimensions of the Warwick and Kelman framework discussed earlier.

In considering the development of a national health insurance system, Jonsen and Butler discuss two moral principles: distributive justice (fair distribution of harms and benefits in society according to standards of equity, desert, need, or contract) and respect for individuals (implying equal treatment for each person who has liberties, rights, and obligations). An example of a discussion between a congressional committee and an ethicist about a national health insurance plan might include several ethical concerns about distributive justice and fairness. Debate about justice and fairness involves the distribution of burdens and benefits to particular socioeconomic groups, whether or not equality is a criterion for distribution, the justification of unequal distribution according to merit or ability, and whether there is an "objective" way to determine a "fair" distribution in terms of the most medically needy (Jonsen & Butler, 1975, p. 28).

In clarifying policy options from an ethical perspective, one must consider the impact of deductibles and coinsurance on the poor, who may be discouraged by them from seeking medical care until their medical conditions are far advanced or they are forced to seek care in an emergency room. Issues of research-supported racial disparities in health care must be considered as well. If relatively small deductibles were paid out of pocket, the public funds "saved" could be used for the patients who must be institutionalized for care. Or, would it be more just to provide "free" preventive and basic care for the very poor and the undocumented people whose health status affects all of us? The ethicist might then show that the criterion of medical need takes priority over the criterion of equality, such as the need arising from poverty or racial disparities, which negatively influence the distribution patterns of illness and disease. From a Rawlsian perspective, one might claim that it is not unfair to improve the position of the least advantaged in our communities. In view of fiscal constraints, is explicit rationing of some types of treatment necessary? One could also argue that it would be more just to establish health policy based on balancing the respective needs of the very sick, the very poor, and the uninsured. Deductibles would vary with income, so that the very poor would pay almost nothing out of pocket. One might also consider equity factors in various proposals for a national health insurance plan in addition to economic consequences, administrative implications, and changes in health care delivery patterns (Jonsen & Butler, 1975, pp. 28–29).

Further ethical considerations that should inform public policy debate about health care were developed in the report of the President's Commission for the *Study of Ethical*

Problems in Medicine and Biomedical and Behavioral Research (1983) on access to health care and in the proposals made by philosopher Daniel Callahan in his book entitled *What Kind of Life: The Limits of Medical Progress* (1989). The President's Commission concluded that society has an ethical obligation to ensure equitable access to health care for all. This ethical obligation rests on the special importance of health care for relief of suffering, prevention of premature death, restoration of functioning, increasing opportunity, provision of information about individual health status, and showing evidence of mutual empathy and compassion (President's Commission, 1983). Additional conclusions related to balancing societal and individual obligations are to share fairly the costs of health care; ensuring that all citizens are able to secure an adequate level of care without excessive burdens; that the ultimate responsibility for ensuring that societal obligations are met rests with the federal government; and that while efforts to contain health care costs are important, they should not focus on limiting access to the most vulnerable population groups in the society (President's Commission, 1983, pp. 4–6). Government, private organizations, and business continue to struggle with what constitutes an adequate level of health care benefits and how to fund them as costs of health care continue to skyrocket. These challenges become even more significant as international travel increases, and there is a corresponding increase in exposure to more communicable diseases.

Callahan's proposals remind us that health is not an end in and of itself (Callahan, 1989). He asserts that health can only have meaning in the context of the overall welfare of our society, that is, the welfare of our social, educational, economic, and cultural institutions. He proposes a different vision of medical progress that gives the highest priority to caring for those who cannot be cured based on a variety of scientific, physiological, or economic realities. No one in need should be abandoned, and individuals should always be treated with compassion as members of the human community. An additional priority would focus on the principles and practices of public health and primary care as they are most conducive to the common good at the least cost. Examples include good nutrition, disease prevention, immunizations, appropriate use of antibiotics, and emergency medicine. Callahan suggests, not uncontroversially, that the last priority for society to pursue in health care is use of advanced forms of high-tech medicine that tend to benefit fewer individuals at comparatively high costs and sometimes add a disproportionate burden to patient suffering. Organ transplants and advanced intensive care services for the very sick elderly are examples. These suggested priorities should guide policy development and implementation according to Callahan. They represent a radical shift from priorities of cure at almost any financial, social, or psychological costs and have profound implications for public and organizational health policy. One can also speculate on where the determination of personal genetic profiles, use of high-tech reproductive procedures, and medical research on use of stem cells for some disease conditions fit in economic, social, and ethical deliberations of public policy for health care financing and delivery.

Allocation of societal resources to health care in relation to the needs of other institutions such as education and social welfare requires some degree of societal consensus about our health goals as the United States now spends over 15 percent of its GDP on health care. Callahan raises the question of whether the search for unlimited medical progress may not lead to the impoverishment of the rest of our lives. He claims that we have drifted along for years "creating a health care system that not only costs too much for what it delivers, but fails also to deliver what it could for millions of people . . . (and) has led us to spend too much on health in comparison with other social needs, too much on the old in comparison with the young, too much on the acutely ill in comparison with the chronically ill, too much on curing in comparison with caring . . . and too much on extending the length of life rather than enhancing the quality of life" (Callahan, 1990).

More recently, the President's Council on Bioethics issued a report entitled *Taking Care: Ethical Caregiving in Our Aging Society* (2005) that incorporates the relationship of policy and "ethical commitments."

The report recognizes the reality that "moral aspirations and moral boundaries— always to care, never to abandon or betray those entrusted to our care—should guide us" as policy is developed in the realities of limited resources and competing social goods (President's Council on Bioethics, 2005). As this report focuses on caregiving for the elderly, we are reminded that government has an obligation to institute ways in which the burden of care is shared more equitably in society so that the elderly and their caregivers will not be abandoned. This obligation rests on ethical values of respect for persons and justice based on equity and need.

Concerns for aging populations and caregiving for the elderly are not limited to the United States. Miriam Hirschfeld, former chief nursing scientist of the World Health Organization (WHO) in Geneva, Switzerland, organized an international effort on the ethics of long-term care. An outcome of the project was a report on issues of justice in long-term care describing caregiver burdens worldwide. Not surprisingly, women were found to bear most of the burdens of care for the elderly around the world (Wikler & Hirschfeld, 2002).

In summary, any comprehensive debate about health policy development and implementation must take into account the ethical values and concerns discussed in this chapter in order to develop ethically supportable policy recommendations that are more than simply attempts to respond to economic and cost considerations. More community-oriented values such as community solidarity and personal security should inform public policy decisions in public, private, and social arenas as an obligation of health care and health-related systems to meet health needs without impoverishment (Priester, 1992b).

FURTHER THOUGHTS FOR NURSING

The nurse collaborates with other health professionals and the public in promoting community, national, and international efforts to meet health needs. And, the profession of nursing, as represented by associations and their members, is responsible for articulating nursing values . . . and for shaping social policy. (*ANA Code of Ethics for Nurses*, 2001)

Meeting nursing's ethical obligations to patients, their families, and communities requires collaboration with health care consumers and their family and social supports, health care professionals, and policy makers, and a reasoned decision-making process in order to shape policy that assures adequate access to health and nursing care. Respect for persons, avoiding harm, and distributive justice are ethical principles that nurses, individually and collectively, can use in reflecting on the interface of ethics and politics in policy development and implementation. The principle of distributive justice requires the fair distribution of burdens and benefits. Burdens include economic costs and human energy costs of care. Provision of needed nursing and health care to promote health goals are benefits. Nurses and others must take issues of justice and other ethical values into account in attempting to meet the health and nursing care needs of individuals, families, and communities through organizational and public policy development and to ensure the survival of organizations to deliver health services.

Nurses and their professional organizations have become more knowledgeable, active, and influential in public policy development and assessment over the past few decades (Mason, Talbott, & Leavitt, 1993). For example, the American Academy of Nursing (AAN) works with a major goal of "advancing health policy" through development of policy-related initiatives and campaigns to spur reform of health care systems using nursing solutions and nurses' expertise.[1] A study, conducted by this author, demonstrated that nurses involved in direct patient care see themselves as a critical resource for legislators and other policymakers in the development of public and institutional policies that affect nursing and patient care (Aroskar, Moldow, & Good, 2004). Indeed, involvement of nurses in policy making was the first recommendation to legislators, along with other key recommendations such as achievement of universal and easy access to health care services and education and development of advocates to assist patients and families to navigate health care systems.

Nursing values of commitment to individuals' right to health care and respect for human dignity are foundational to nurses' involvement in health policy development (Davis, 1988). Medical and nursing needs, as determined increasingly by research, support policy for distribution of health care benefits and for perspectives on rights to and obligations in health care. If these needs are not met, people suffer and are unable to carry out their life plans and activities. Needs may be considered on a spectrum extending from needs that arise in the individual such as those created by life-threatening illness, through needs for prevention of disease, to needs that arise from unhealthy environments Health-related needs that arise in and from the environment include provision of potable water, safe food supplies, safe working conditions, and clean air. Assurance of healthy environments is required for human survival and flourishing. At the same time, health and health-related needs compete with other social needs and interests, such as public safety and education, for limited public resources.

Health policy development and implementation are continuing challenges to nursing's ethics and values even as nurses can and are taking leadership to articulate such needs in policy making in institutional and governmental arenas, supported by the *ANA Code of Ethics for Nurses* (2001). While these efforts continue, the needs of the uninsured or underinsured still go unmet and continue to have social and economic consequences for our society. While managed care arrangements represent a major restructuring of health care services and their financing, such plans generally consider their goals and obligations to be meeting needs of members and containing costs.

There are several decisions that individual nurses, groups of nurses, and professional nursing organizations can make related to participation in policy development:

1. Decisions about the types of public or private health and health-related organizations and at what level (local, state, national, or international) they will participate
2. Types of participation—ranging from financial support for groups working on goals supported by nursing and personal values to active participation in policy-making bodies

3. Whether or not the nursing profession will take even stronger initiatives in developing ethically responsible and responsive health policy in health care organizations and in government arenas.

Specific actions in the ethical domain related to policy development, implementation, and assessment of existing policy include:

1. Examining the goals of existing or proposed policies
2. Clearly identifying the persons or groups who are the actual or proposed targets of policy change and their participation in policy processes
3. Identifying the underlying ethical assumptions of policy
4. Discussing the methods proposed to implement policy
5. Assessing the short- and long-term consequences of policy proposals or changes to the greatest degree possible
6. Identifying the ethical principles and values that are at stake in policy proposals and changes with use of the *ANA Code of Ethics for Nurses* (2001) as one resource among others.

Taking such specific actions can lead to the development of an ethical impact statement similar to an environmental impact statement that may lead to different policy decisions from those that occur without such reflection and discussion.

Acting in the spirit of "preventive ethics" integrated with sensitivity to political power considerations will not lead automatically to one ethically acceptable set of decisions or policies. Such analysis *will* rule out policy proposals that completely ignore the impact of a proposed policy on respect for individual autonomy or equity in access to health care for the most vulnerable (Aroskar, 1987). It is a moral imperative that the impact of proposed and existing health policies on the sickest individuals, the dying, pregnant women, children, ethnic minorities, and the poverty-stricken always be taken seriously as considerations of justice, caring, and human rights.

Nurses, as patient advocates and citizens, can and should become more knowledgeable about the interaction of social, ethical, legal, economic, and political aspects of institutional and public policy decisions as one form of power. Numerous opportunities are available to learn about health and health-related policy through policy concentrations in graduate nursing programs, onsite and online courses, and through policy-focused conferences. These educational experiences will assist nurses who seek to influence policy decisions individually and collectively through professional organizations or other community groups in both public and private sectors. Choosing to do nothing about health policy development and implementation is a choice that has consequences for the nursing profession and its care populations. Making ethically responsible decisions for policy action requires a reexamination of values underlying the rhetoric of nursing and the behavior of nurses, individually and collectively. An exclusive focus on care of individual patients and their families, while still the *sine qua non* of nursing care delivery, is not adequate by itself for the societal role and moral obligations of professional nursing in our turbulent times of radical world-wide change and uncertainty. The claim that nurses are patient advocates points to an obligation to participate and provide leadership in institutional and public policy making and development of adequate systems of care and education for current and future patients and patient populations.

The tasks involved in the development of ethically responsible policy are difficult and complex. They require the critical thinking and leadership of nurses and others in health care systems that affect and are affected by delivery of nursing care. A sense of powerlessness and moral distress in nursing often leads to inaction rather than the leadership necessary to meet patient and societal needs for nursing and health care. Such realities pose tremendous challenges to the integrity of the profession, to nursing education, and to all organizations that provide nursing services in acute care, long-term care, psychiatric care, home care, prisons, schools, the military, and the workplace. Nurses, in the study mentioned earlier, were *most* concerned that they were compromised in the ability to meet their ethical obligations to patients and families as governmental and workplace policies changed without nursing input (Aroskar, Moldow, & Good, 2004).

Responses to these challenges must include an explicit focus on identification and clarification of ethical values in health care delivery arrangements such as service and compassion that should guide individual and organizational behaviors (Norling & Pashley, 1995; Reiser, 1994). The Joint Commission on Accreditation of Healthcare Organizations (2008) has required attention to patient rights and responsibilities and the development of a code of ethics for organizational behavior as a requirement for accreditation for more than a decade. This requirement has led to an emphasis on organizational ethics and development of plans that provide ways to respond to ethical issues in patient care and related services. These include institutional ethics committees, more attention to the ethical practices of health care organizations, and availability of ethics consultants.

Ethical obligations of the nursing profession in practice, education, research, and policy development are articulated in its ethical codes. As nurses and citizens, we are challenged to participate in developing health policies reflective of identified ethical values that are individually, professionally, environmentally, and socially oriented. These are essential considerations in making more holistic decisions about the allocation of finite resources at all levels of government and in health service and other health-related organizations. While such deliberations are not easy in today's competitive and radically changing health care systems, such reflection and action are vital to meeting nursing's social mandate. Organizational, national, and international health policies affect all of us as interconnected and interdependent individuals and affect the environments in which we live, work, and play around the world.

CASE STUDY I

You have been asked to serve as a nursing representative on a government committee to look at funding for health care of undocumented individuals who work in the United States. You are well aware that a comprehensive immigration bill has yet to be developed and that these individuals are working in the country as illegal immigrants. Ethical requirements to provide health care for those in need conflict with legal and political realities. At the same time, you know that health conditions of everyone in society affect all individuals and families who reside in communities legally or illegally. Undocumented workers and their children are in the workplace, schools, stores, banks, and other venues where people gather.

Suggested Questions for Discussion

1. What professional nursing values should be considered when developing the committee's response?
2. What are the goals of the proposed policy or policy options?
3. Who or what is expected to change in the proposed policy, e.g., patient or provider behaviors?
4. What are the means or methods selected to implement the policy and how are they justified ethically?
5. What are some of the direct and indirect consequences for individuals, organizations, and the community if the committee recommends that no public funding be provided for health care of undocumented people working in the United States?
6. What help is provided for you in the *ANA Code of Ethics for Nurses* (2001) in reflecting on the elements of the policy proposal or policy options being considered by the committee?

CASE STUDY II

You have been asked to serve as the nursing representative on an environmental health committee in your county. There have been several cases of childhood leukemia in the county and the environmental health committee has been asked to respond to conflicting evidence that has recently been published for carcinogen levels in both air and water in your county. These levels are being attributed to mining companies and waste disposal sites in your county and surrounding counties after this evidence has been published in local newspapers. At the same time, you are aware of funding deficits in the counties and the state as well as federal mandates for environmental clean-up that may or may not have federal funds attached to them.

Suggested Questions for Discussion

1. What are the ethical nursing values that may be challenged for you as the nursing representative on the committee?
2. What are the goals in developing a policy response for this situation?
3. Who or what are the potential targets of change in developing a policy response for this situation?
4. What means or methods are chosen to develop a policy response and how are they justified ethically?
5. What are the direct and indirect consequences or "costs" for the individuals, groups, and communities identified as targets of change?
6. What help is provided for you in the *ANA Code of Ethics for Nurses* (2001) in reflecting on the conflicting evidence and development of a policy response to the situation described in this case study?

Notes

1. For details on the American Academy of Nursing (AAN) policy and policy-related activities, check website www.aannet.org/policy

References

American Nurses Association. (2001). *Code of ethics for nurses with interpretive statements.* Washington, DC: American Nurses Association Publishing.

American Nurses Association. (2005). *ANA's Health Care Agenda-2005.* Washington, DC: American Nurses Association Publishing.

Aroskar, M. A. (1987). The interface of ethics and politics in nursing. *Nursing Outlook, 37*(6), 268–272.

Aroskar, M. A., Moldow, D. G., & C. M. Good (2004). Nurses' voices: Policy, practice, and ethics. *Nursing Ethics, 11*(3), 274.

Callahan, D. (1989). *What kind of life? The limits of medical progress.* New York: Simon & Schuster.

Callahan, D. (1990). Modernizing mortality: Medical progress and the good society. *Hastings Center Report, 20*(1), 28–32.

The Center for Biomedical Ethics. (1989). *Rethinking medical morality: The ethical implications of changes in health care organization, delivery, and financing.* Minneapolis: University of Minnesota.

Chapman, C. B., & Talmadge, J. M. (1971). The evolution of the right to health concept in United States. *Pharos, 34*, 31–33.

Davis, G. C. (1988). Nursing values and health care policy. *Nursing Outlook, 36*(6), 289–292.

Fuchs, V. R. (1974). *Who shall live?* New York: Basic Books.

Jonsen, A. R., & Butler, L. H. (1975). Public ethics and policy making. *Hastings Center Report, 5*(4), 19–31.

Kalisch, B. J., & Kalisch, P. A. (1982). *Politics of nursing.* Philadelphia: Lippincott.

Mason, D. J., Talbott, S. W., & Leavitt, J. K. (1993). *Policy and politics for nurses* (2nd ed.). Philadelphia: W. B. Saunders.

Norling, R. A., & Pashley, S. (1995). Identifying and strengthening core values. *Managed Care Quarterly, 3*, 11–28.

President's Commission for the Study of Ethical Problems in Medicine and Biomedical and Behavioral Research. (1983). *Securing access to health care,* Report Vol. 1. Washington, DC: Government Printing Office, p. 4.

President's Council on Bioethics. (2005). *Taking care: Ethical caregiving in our aging society* (pp. 208–209). Washington, DC.

Priester, R. (1990). Health-care values buried by cost-control emphasis. *Minnesota Journal, 7*, 1.

Priester, R. (1992a). A values framework for health system reform. *Health Affairs, 11*(1), 84–107.

Priester, R. (1992b). A values framework for health system reform. *Health Affairs, 11*(2), 84–107.

Reiser, S. J. (1994). The ethical life of health care organizations. *Hastings Center Report, 24*(6), 28–35.

Stevens, R. (1971). *American medicine and the public interest.* New Haven: Yale University Press.

Strickland, S. P. (1972). *Politics, science, and dread disease.* Cambridge, MA: Harvard University.

Warwick, K. D., & Kelman, H. C. (1976). Ethical issues in social intervention. In W. G. Bennis, K. D. Benne, R. Chin, et al. (Eds.), *The planning of change* (3rd ed., p. 470). New York: Holt, Rinehart, & Winston.

Wikler, D., & Hirschfeld, M. (Eds.). (June 2002). *Ethical choices in long term care: What does justice require?* Geneva: World Health Organization.

Wilson, F. A., & Neuhauser, D. (1982). *Health services in the United States* (2nd ed.). Cambridge, MA: Ballinger.

CHAPTER 11

Where to Next: Gathering the Issues

Whether because of need or of curiosity, the world skitters about on its own unrest. Science and technology change; culture changes; even the world changes. What is unchanging is that ethical assessments and decisions will continue to need to be made. How then are we to confront the ethical issues on the near and far horizon? Scientific and technological advance will bring new clinical knowledge and interventions, but may not raise new ethical issues. Changes in national demographics will bring new cultural understandings that may not raise new ethical issues, but may challenge the ways in which we understand old ones. Changes in the world that have made it "smaller" and that have made health more "global" and less insular may not raise new ethical issues, but may bring worldwide issues to our doorstep. On the other hand, all of these changes may in fact raise new issues. How are we to think about and anticipate these changes and the ethical demands that they make?

CHANGES IN SCIENCE AND TECHNOLOGY

Of all of the exciting advances in bioscience, none excite the imagination quite so much as those associated with the mapping of the human genome. The project of mapping the human genome began in 1990 and was completed in 2003. The project goals were to

- *identify* all the approximately 20,000–25,000 genes in human DNA,
- *determine* the sequences of the 3 billion chemical base pairs that make up human DNA,
- *store* this information in databases,
- *improve* tools for data analysis,
- *transfer* related technologies to the private sector, and
- *address* the ethical, legal, and social issues (ELSI) that may arise from the project.[1]

Along the way, the project also involved mapping the genes of *E. coli*, the fruit fly, and the laboratory mouse. This government-sponsored project gave rise to the new field of *genomics*. Genomics is "the scientific study of genomes, using gene mapping, nucleotide sequencing, and other techniques; the branch of molecular biology concerned with the structure, function, and evolution of genomes" (Simpson & Weiner, 1989).

The hopes that the project raises are for more accurate diagnosis and prediction of disease and specific disease susceptibility and for more targeted and effective disease prevention and intervention. More specifically, the project raises the intriguing possibility of a genetically based, individualized medicine for both prevention and treatment of disease. Researchers are moving toward identifying the genetic components of disease in groups of persons as well as in particular individuals.

Breast cancer serves as a good example here. Not all breast cancers are the same. Two tumor-suppressor genes have been identified for breast cancer: BRCA1 (breast cancer gene 1) and BRCA2. When they function normally, these genes help prevent tumor development by repairing damaged DNA. In 1994, it was discovered that women who have mutations of BRCA1 or BRCA2 have a higher risk of developing breast and ovarian cancer. HER2/neu (human epidermal growth factor receptor 2) is another gene that regulates cell growth and is responsible for the pathogenesis of particularly aggressive breast cancer. When the HER2 gene is altered, additional HER2 receptors are produced, leading to increased cell growth and reproduction and more aggressive tumor cells. In addition, researchers have discovered a p53 gene tumor suppressor that, when mutated, also increases a woman's risk of developing breast cancer. Currently, this information allows clinicians to predict the clinical course of a specific breast cancer and to predict which treatments will be more and which less effective for a given breast cancer. Genetic testing results can indicate an increased risk for breast cancer and, depending upon the specific gene mutation found, signal a need for regular breast self-exam, more frequent mammograms, possible chemoprevention, possibly even prophylactic mastectomy. The hope of genetic-based care is, of course, the development of drugs that target specific genes, thus tailoring chemoprevention or chemotherapy to the individual's particular gene mutation or susceptibility. The U.S. Food and Drug Administration (FDA) has approved the drug Herceptin® (trastuzumab). Clinical trials have shown that Herceptin can slow the growth and spread of cancerous tumors in women who are HER2 positive. As knowledge of cancer genetics advances, it will help to identify at-risk individuals earlier, establish individualized treatment regimens precisely aimed at molecular levels of the disease, and lead to the development of new drugs for specific cancer genetic types (Lindor, Lindor, & Greene, 2006). Thus, genetic medicine has implications for cancer screening, prevention, and treatment. As in the mythical "Old West," where the lawman had a bullet with the crook's name on it, genodrugs will become bullets with the specific cancer's name on it.

Genomics holds another promise: the potential for using genes themselves to treat or perhaps cure hereditary or acquired genetic diseases by using normal genes to replace, supplement, or repair defective ones or to increase immunity to specific diseases. What is now science fiction, the in utero treatment and cure of hereditary diseases such as cystic fibrosis, no longer looks like an impossibility. It is an exciting prospect that some devastating hereditary genetic diseases such as Tay-Sachs disease, muscular dystrophies, cystic fibrosis, sickle-cell disease, and cri du chat could be eradicated. Genetic treatment could even be used to affect hereditary conditions not considered diseases, such as color blindness, male-pattern baldness, or type of ear wax. There are two genetically determined types of ear wax: wet and dry. Dry ear wax is associated with Native American and Asian peoples (Overfield, 1985). Ear wax types have been used by anthropologists to track human migratory patterns, such as those of the Inuit. The genetic type that produces dry ear wax also causes reduced sweat production that, it is conjectured by researchers, was beneficial to the Native Americans and Asians who lived in cold climates (Bass & Jackson, 1977; Yoshiura *et al.*, 2006). While genomics can revolutionize medical treatment, it can also produce developments in many other fields such as anthropology.

Genetic research will also uncover information beyond diseases, such as the genetics of food preferences or food intolerances. Is there any truth to the "genotype diet" that links specific foods to be eaten to one's blood type (D'Adamo, 2007)? Advances in genomics should help us sort out a wide range of claims of this nature. Genomics is making strides in studies of specific populations. For example, Native Americans of North America and indigenous people of Oceania are susceptible to what is called *New World Syndrome* (Harris & Ross, 1987). New World Syndrome is thought to have a genetic component that leads to an enhanced ability to store fat. More specifically, there are several genetic factors that bring about the conversion of some carbohydrates into adenosine triphosphate (ATP) more efficiently than in other populations. It is hypothesized that this ability developed as a consequence of the cycles of famine to which Native American peoples historically were subject. This ability, in turn, leads to a higher than expected rate of obesity, heart disease, diabetes, hypertension, and shorter life span among Native Americans who stray from their traditional to a "modern" diet.[2] Genetic studies ultimately may have a good deal to contribute to our understanding of, for instance, the interactions of my own diet, exercise, and my health and sense of bodily well-being.

What are the moral issues that are raised by these advances in genomics? Despite the astonishing potential for new approaches to disease prevention and treatment, many of the issues that genomics raises are "something old," not "something new." The same "old" ethical issues that are raised by current laboratory or diagnostic tests in general are also raised by emerging patient genetic studies: privacy (Rothstein, 1997), confidentiality, labeling, stigmatization, and discrimination. Large social issues that have been raised in the past in discussion of mental illness or developmental disabilities resurface with genomics. These questions include the following:

- reproductive rights: who has the legal/social right to reproduce and to perpetuate defective genes?
- social Darwinism or eugenics: the right of society to "engineer" its gene pool for the betterment of society through both "negative eugenics" (e.g., involuntary sterilization) and "positive eugenics" (e.g., prenatal testing, screening, and treatment; pre-pregnancy genetic testing and counseling; genetic engineering, in vitro and through other reproductive technologies)
- normative understandings of humankind: what is a "normal," "healthy," "productive," person or what is the range of normal that is acceptable to society?
- philosophical questions of what it means to be human: what is "human," what is "person," or "personhood," and what is the relationship between person and society?

Many of these issues have been discussed elsewhere in this book. However, it is useful to revisit a representative patient issue. Consider the case of Terri Seargent. In 1999, she went to her physician with a complaint of breathing difficulties. Genetic testing revealed that she had alpha-1 antitrypsin deficiency. This disorder in its severe form leads to early onset emphysema (in the 30s or 40s), disability, and reduced life expectancy and may necessitate lung and liver transplant. Early detection meant that Ms. Seargent could receive life-saving treatment. However, this is a costly condition and when her employer learned of the results of her test, she was fired and lost her health insurance. It is called "genetic discrimination." There is increasing evidence that employers have engaged in genetic discrimination and hired and fired on the basis of genetic tests (Martindale, 2001). Increasingly, federal and state laws are being promulgated to obstruct genetic discrimination. Who should have access to information from genetic testing and ethically, how may it be used? This question is an old question for occupational health nurses; employers want information that will reduce their costs—whether related to health care insurance or to employee training and retention costs. But employers are not the only ones who want this information. Insurers, schools, adoption agencies, courts, the military, and other social agencies all want this information for their own purposes. Those purposes rarely redound to the benefit of the person who has been tested. Nurses, however, are not agents of society, primarily serving the interests of society or the common good. Neither are they primarily agents of an employer. The ANA *Code of Ethics for Nurses* (2001) is crystal clear: "The Nurse's primary commitment is to the patient, whether an individual, group, or community" (American Nurses Association, 2001). Davis notes that

> Historically, nurses had ethical obligations that placed emphasis on attending to the patient's needs, and yet the context of nursing was not necessarily supportive of this obligation. Today, the nurse's ethical obligation to the patient, first, is even more complex to negotiate . . . . nurses must deal with economic pressures that may compete with moral values or with patient's rights. The patients and their rights must remain central. (Davis, 2008)

Genomics raises larger social issues as well, issues that we have also seen before. In the famous case *Buck v Bell* (1927),[3] the U.S. Supreme Court upheld a Virginia statue for compulsory sterilization for the mentally retarded, specifically for the purpose of eugenics, that is, for the purpose of improving the human gene pool. The case centered on Carrie Buck, an 18-year-old inmate of Virginia State Colony for Epileptics and Feebleminded. The state sought to have her sterilized. She was the daughter of a woman with a record of prostitution and immorality, and Carrie herself was deemed to be "feebleminded." Carrie gave birth to an illegitimate child. Her adopted family had her committed as feebleminded with the taint of immorality. As it was later discovered, Carrie's "immorality" was the consequence of rape by the nephew of the adopted family and her commitment was an attempt to preserve the family's reputation. The ruling was written by Justice Oliver Wendell Holmes, Jr. In support of his argument that the interest of the states in a "pure" gene pool outweighed the interest of individuals in their bodily integrity, he argued

> We have seen more than once that the public welfare may call upon the best citizens for their lives. It would be strange if it could not call upon those who already sap the strength of the State for these lesser sacrifices, often not felt to be such by those concerned, in order to prevent our being

swamped with incompetence. It is better for all the world, if instead of waiting to execute degenerate offspring for crime, or to let them starve for their imbecility, society can prevent those who are manifestly unfit from continuing their kind. The principle that sustains compulsory vaccination is broad enough to cover cutting the Fallopian tubes.[4]

In arguing for genetic purity and for removing the genetically unfit from participation in the gene pool, Holmes concluded his argument with the infamous statement, "Three generations of imbeciles are enough."[5]

The United States has an approximately 150-year history of attempting to genetically engineer society to control undesirable social behaviors (e.g., criminality, seafaringness, vagrancy, prostitution, and immorality) and perpetuate desirable behaviors and attributes (e.g., intelligence, reduced suffering, and general human improvement). One can see the extreme of where this can lead: the "racial hygiene" of the Nazi Holocaust. Our history has been based on a fairly primitive genetic science. Imagine the potential for engineering society with an advanced genetic technology. The possibilities would range from the eradication of specific diseases and hereditary conditions to designing future generations of one's family. "Negative eugenics" could also be implemented by prohibiting procreation among those whose "defects" could not be controlled.

The moral and philosophical questions that are raised by these potentials are substantial. *Disease* and *health* are social constructs as much as they are biological conditions. This means that what counts as a *disease* or *health* is defined by society and goes beyond what is biologically based. For instance, the WHO definition of health greatly exceeds biology: "Health is a state of complete physical, mental, and social well-being and not merely the absence of disease or infirmity" (World Health Organization, 1946). Subsequent revision of the definition states that "health is a resource for everyday life, not the objective of living," and "health is a positive concept emphasizing social and personal resources, as well as physical capacities" (World Health Organization, 1986).

What then is a disease and what shall we treat? Huntington's is a disease. Is color-blindness, left-handedness, a widow's peak, curved thumb, attached ear lobes, longer second toe, middle knuckle hair, or being very short or very tall a disease?

Society is built around a normative understanding of the human person. One only needs to be shorter than normal, taller than normal, or left-handed to recognize the existence of certain presuppositions about what is "normal." Each of us has an idea of what is "normal," though we do not often reflect upon this. Just as it is important for patient care that nurses reflect upon what they think about death, dying, sex, and religion, it is equally important for nurses to understand their own normative view of humans. That normative view will then influence what the nurse might regard as acceptable, repugnant, beautiful, handicapped, admirable, deviant, and so on. Chapter 9 on mental illness and developmental disability raises the issue of how individual nurses feel about those with developmental disabilities, specifically those with conditions that are socially disvalued. The potential of genetic science expands that consideration to include not only what society finds a disvalue (and would seek to control), but also what society values in persons and how that might attempt to be engineered or implemented in genetic manipulation in the future. Then, with the potential of genetic engineering, how might society treat those who would choose not to participate, to opt out? How might society choose to treat those who did have disabilities of one sort or another. Might society even choose to produce classes of servant individuals who might be less intellectually capable? Might individuals be held responsible individually, and denied or given access to health care, for eating/not eating those foods linked to their genetics? Imagine being arrested and incarcerated for eating a burger instead of squash and beans. Novel after novel has creatively raised such questions, sometimes in quite alarming scenarios. While such engineering remains in the speculative future, it is important for nurses to engage in the *Gedankenexperiment*, the thought experiment, of how they might respond if such engineering were a reality, and what social policies they might support. More specifically, it is important for nurses to consider questions such as these:

- What is my normative understanding of human persons?
- What kind of society ought we to be with regard to those who are ill, declining, frail, disabled, or who suffer from traumatic injury?
- What social policies do I believe should or should not be implemented in striving for human well-being and human flourishing?
- To what extent should medicine and nursing be used to achieve social goals?

At the same time, it is crucial to remember the words of the *Code of Ethics for Nurses*: "The nurse, in all professional relationships, practices with compassion and respect for the inherent worth, dignity, and human rights of every individual. Nurses take into account the needs and values of all persons in all professional relationships" (ANA, 2001).

Most technological and scientific advances carry both promise and threat, hope and fears. It is encouraging that the Human Genome Project had as a key aspect of the project research on ethical, legal, and social issues. The project information includes the following statement:

> A continuing challenge is to safeguard the privacy of individuals and groups who contribute DNA samples for large-scale sequence-variation studies. Other concerns have been to anticipate how the resulting data may affect concepts of race and ethnicity; identify potential uses (or misuses) of genetic data in workplaces, schools, and courts; identify commercial uses; and foresee impacts of genetic advances on the concepts of humanity and personal responsibility.[6]

Part of "getting it right" requires that scientists, researchers, and practitioners inextricably link their work with a consideration of the ethical issues that are raised. Science at its best is ethical science.

CHANGES IN SOCIETY

Ethical issues in health care do not arise solely from science and technology. The very nature of society itself and its cultural patterns also raise ethical issues. Structural injustices have long been of concern to nursing. Specifically, injustices that have led to limited or no access to health care and nursing have been of concern to nursing for decades. The eighth provision of the *Code of Ethics for Nurses* states, "The nurse collaborates with other health professionals and the public in promoting community, national and international efforts to meet health needs" (ANA, 2001). This is an activist stance that is reinforced by the interpretive statement:

> The nursing profession is committed to promoting the health, welfare and safety of all people. The nurse has a responsibility to be aware not only of specific needs of individual patient but also of broader health concerns such as world hunger, environmental pollution, lack of access to health care, violation of human rights, and inequitable distribution of nursing and health care resources. The availability and accessibility of high quality health services to all people require both interdisciplinary planning and collaborative partnerships among health professionals and others at the community, national, and international levels. (ANA, 2001)

This is a concern for justice and social policy/health policy and is the subject of heated national debate, especially in election years. But there is more to this discussion, more that comes closer to the practicing nurse.

Let's go back to eugenics for a moment. The United States has a history of laws enforcing racial segregation publicly and privately through "anti-miscegenation" laws (from Latin *miscêre* to mix + *genus* race) (Simpson & Weiner, 1989) that prohibited interracial marriage. Such laws pre-dated the eugenics movement; the colony of Virginia instituted a law prohibiting interracial marriage between Blacks and Whites in 1691. Many of the states had such laws until, in 1967, the Virginia law was overturned as unconstitutional. But, who was Black and who was White? Some states had laws nicknamed "one drop laws," by which even a single drop of Black blood resulted in being categorized as Black. Later anti-miscegenation and anti-incest laws were justified on eugenic grounds.

Stephen J. Gould and others have maintained that immigration laws such as the Immigration Act of 1924 and the Immigration and Nationality Act of 1965 have been motivated by the eugenic goals of preventing the immigration of "inferior stock" and maintaining the dominance and superiority of White, Western European Americans (Gould, 1981). Others have argued that the concerns for the restriction of immigration have been based on a desire to preserve the cultural purity of the nation against the ingress of foreign cultures (Herrnstein, 1983). In either case, significant interracial and intercultural tensions and prejudices persist in the United States at a time when immigration patterns have brought increasing numbers of nurses and patients from other countries and cultures into the health care system. Currently, approximately 12 percent of the U.S. nursing workforce is foreign born and foreign educated (Nichols, 2007). In addition, there are approximately one million immigrants (including "change of status" immigrants already in the United States). There are over 37 million legal immigrants in the United States and there will be an estimated increase of 1.5 million illegal immigrants per year in addition to the estimated 12–20 million illegal immigrants already here. There has been an increase of 57% in the foreign-born population in the United States between 1990 and 2000 (Gibson & Lennon, 1999).[7] Thus, approximately 12 percent of the nurses and 12 percent of the population are foreign born, though there are higher numbers of persons not foreign born who are strongly affiliated with language or culture-based communities within the United States. Some states receive much higher numbers of immigrants. For example, in California, one in four residents is an immigrant. By 1995, almost 33 percent of the nation's immigrants resided in California (Vernez & McCarthy, 1997).

Immigration holds a number of implications for health care, not the least of which is that of access to care and the cost of care. However, immigration affects the nurse and nursing practice more intimately when the nurse meets with a patient whose culture and perhaps language do not represent that of the nurse. World cultures are rife with health beliefs and practices that are not necessarily shared with other cultures. Even more importantly for this discussion, there are profound cultural differences in the interpretation of ethical norms—differences of which the nurse must be aware. The *Code of Ethics for Nurses*, interpretive statement 1.2, states:

> The need for health care is universal, transcending all individual differences. The nurse establishes relationships and delivers nursing services with respect for human needs and values, without prejudice. Such consideration does not suggest that the nurse necessarily agrees with or condones certain individual choices, but that the nurse respects the patient as a person. (ANA, 2001)

Values and the ethical decisions that develop from those values are embedded in culture, interpreted through the lens of culture, and shared within culture. Cultural diversity is an essential and enriching aspect of humanity's condition. The UNESCO Universal Declaration on Cultural Diversity notes this:

> Culture takes diverse forms across time and space. This diversity is embodied in the uniqueness and plurality of the identities of the groups and societies making up humankind. As a source of exchange, innovation and creativity, cultural diversity is as necessary for humankind as biodiversity is for nature. In this sense, it is the common heritage of humanity and should be recognized and affirmed for the benefit of present and future generations. (UNESCO, 2002)

Cultural diversity demands of us that we look through the eyes of others and not only through our own eyes. Nurses must attempt to understand as the patient understands and to affirm the patient's values and decisions. This necessitates some "adjustments" to our understanding of ethics.

A number of cultural studies can inform our understanding of culture. For instance, Edward Hall maintains that there are "high-context cultures" and "low-context cultures" (Hall, 1989). In high-context cultures, information either is in the physical context or is internalized in the members of the group. Little is explicit in the transmitted part of the language. In high-context cultures, tradition, unity, harmony, and community are high values and maintain the close social bondedness. Considerable body language may have a common meaning, and they may "talk around" a subject, discussing it without ever discussing it directly. In low-context cultures, on the other hand, the explicit verbal message, whether written or oral, is highly valued as a means of communication. Persons of low-context cultures are often less aware of their cultures or assume that they are culture neutral. They look for "universal rules" in interactions and do not make a great distinction between "insiders" and "outsiders" in the culture. High-context cultures prefer indirect, ambiguous, cautious, nonconfrontational, and subtle ways of communication and of sorting out relationship tangles. Face-saving tactful resolution is sought. Persons from low-context cultures are more likely to engage in direct and one-to-one confrontation (Hall, 1989). The implications of these cultural differences for "informed consent," communication of unhappy diagnoses, and more should be clear, perhaps painfully clear. American law advances a low-context cultural set of norms. To some degree, so does American bioethics. Picture this conversation:

X: Did you tell her that she has cancer? She has a right to know.

Y: Well, yes. But not in so many words.

X: What do you mean "but not in so many words"? Did you tell her or not?

Y: Well yes, I told her without telling her, so she knows.

And around it goes. Can a person be told unequivocally that she has cancer without ever uttering the words "you have cancer"? Of course. For high-context cultures, the indirectness of communication ought to be preserved—and utilized.

Hofstede identifies multiple cultural differences, including power distance, uncertainty avoidance, individualism versus collectivism, and masculinity versus femininity (Hofstede, 2003). *Power distance* refers to the extent to which society accepts the fact that power in institutions and organizations is distributed unequally. In high power distance cultures, there is a belief that there should be and is an order to power. Inequalities in power are accepted as natural and inevitable. Power holders are responsible for looking after the powerless and for providing supervision. Low power distance cultures focus on equality of status and the reduction of power differentials. The willingness of a patient to be "assertive" in securing information or in participating in (or refusing to participate in) decisions regarding care can be culturally conditioned. Some patients may expect the nurse or the physician to "do what they think is best," a position that tends to make nurses recoil. Nurses are taught the value of "self-care" and the patient's right to self-determination. However, we tend not to think of the right to self-determination as a right not to participate. Sometimes, patient self-determination resides in declining to participate in decision making—however uncomfortable that may make us feel.

As another simple example of the way in which culture may attenuate our understanding of ethics, we turn to individualist versus collectivist cultures. Individualist cultures give priority to personal goals, individual identity, the fulfillment of one's potential, assertion of one's strength, separation from others (individuation), and respect for one's physical and psychological space. By contrast, in collectivist cultures, decisions are not made on one's own but in consultation with family or group members, taking into account family or group interests. Well-being and harmony of the group come first. Each person belongs to the community of shared values, beliefs, and traditions, and decisions are embraced by the community (Hofstede, 2003).

As an example of the way in which culture must be considered in clinical ethics, let us look at Native Americans, specifically the Dakota. Scemons writes that

> For any Native American or more largely for Native American traditions and
> even for Indigenous Peoples overall, the written word has limited or no
> meaning. The Native American and Dakota traditions are rooted in oral
> history and tradition, passed orally from generation-to-generation across

the centuries. The spoken word "always has precedence over the written word." The lesser importance of the written word to a modern day Native American of Dakota lineage is based on both collective experience and a fundamental spiritual understanding. . . . More importantly, the written word is of lesser import to Native and Dakota persons because it does not have the same spiritual origin as the spoken word. (Scemons, 2006)

Native cultures generally, and Dakota culture specifically, are communitarian, high context, and nonconfrontational, employing indirect communication. Decisions often await the arrival of the community at the bedside and are collectively made and affirmed. Communicating information requires very cautious, carefully chosen words, perhaps directed toward the whole of the community present, and in some instances, foregoing a written consent in favor of documentation of consent given verbally. In this context, autonomy is exercised by the community as a whole, not by the individual.

When nurses face caring for a patient or patients of a culture not their own, there are several questions that nurses must ask of themselves. These questions include the following:

- What do I know about this culture regarding health-related beliefs and practices?
- What do I need to know of this culture in order to give high-quality nursing care?
- How does my cultural style of communication differ from the patient's?
- What are my cultural or racial or ethnic prejudices, and how might they affect my practice in general, and with this specific patient?
- How do I feel about immigrants, documented or undocumented?

In addition, when working with colleagues of different cultures, nurses must ask the following:

- What are my attitudes toward foreign-born, foreign-educated nurses?
- What are my attitudes toward U.S.-born, U.S.-educated nurses?
- What are my biases and prejudices when working with nurses of a culture or nationality different from my own?
- What are my biases and prejudices toward specific cultures?
- What do I need to know about my colleagues' culture in order to work collaboratively for optimal patient care and for effective teamwork?

Brief though this discussion may be, it serves to caution nurses that increasing cultural diversity as a consequence of immigration, particularly in the Southern border, Atlantic, and Pacific Rim states, is required for morally sensitive practice. Nursing has always affirmed the need to take into account the personal attributes of the patient in planning care. Those differences must also be taken into account when examining the moral understandings of patients who represent a rich and challenging diversity of cultures.

CHANGES IN THE WORLD

Instant worldwide communications, wars and genocide, global mobility and migration, economic and trade agreements, cooperative programs such as the space station, global warming, and much, much more have changed our world and have affected health in many different ways. The butterfly effect, usually applied in chaos theory and science fiction accounts of time travel, has some relevance to our discussion of health. The butterfly effect says that minor, ordinary actions (such as the flap of a single butterfly's wings in a distant part of the world) can result in major, concatenating, and widespread effects in the future (such as a tornado in a distant place). The screen films *It's a Wonderful Life* (1946), *Back to the Future II* (1989), *Frequency* (2000), and the *Terminator* film series (1984–2003) all demonstrate the butterfly effect. How might the butterfly effect influence health and disease? Hirschfield, quoting Friedman, notes that:

> Globalization resulted from worldwide integration of economic and financial sectors. This development was made possible by technological progress . . . geopolitical changes . . . and the dominant ideology of regulation by the market. It has resulted in a phenomenon illustrated by an anecdote a well known journalist relates. A Bangkok taxi driver told him "when you sneeze in New York, I catch a cold." (Hirschfield, 2006)

Hirschfield continues:

> The reality of globalization has considerable impact on nurses' daily work. International travel and trade bring us within weeks of the viruses and bacteria from far away, with SARS being a recent vivid example. International terror exports fear and injuries with new infringements on civil liberties. All these realities affect our health, our need for health services and the way nurses work. (Hirschfield, 2006)

Some global health consequences are less direct than the travel of viruses and bacteria. For example, increased greenhouse gas emissions from fuel combustion (e.g., from power plants, cars, and industry) result in increasing desertification, an expansion of the world's deserts, making the land unsuitable for agriculture and causing population migration to urban areas and often to urban slums (United Nations Convention to Combat Desertification, 2004). In addition, rising sea levels due to polar cap melting threaten polar animals (such as polar bears) as well as persons living on islands in the South Pacific Ocean. The Tuvalu Islands and the Maldives are at imminent risk for loss of their total landmass, and ancestral home, from rising seas. Potentially, approximately 325,000 persons could become refugees from these islands. The inhabitants of Tuvalu Islands, suffering severe flooding of their islands, encroachment of the sea into their fresh water supply, loss of agricultural land, and a rise in the number of fierce cyclones have asked Australia for permission to immigrate but were denied. They have asked New Zealand to accept their 11,000 inhabitants but have received no response as yet (Brown, 2001). Resettlement of refugees has become a problem worldwide.

Wars too cause worldwide changes in health. The U.S.-led war in Iraq has led to more than two million Iraqi refugees. The *Washington Post* notes that:

> Nearly 2 million Iraqis—about 8 percent of the prewar population—have embarked on a desperate migration, mostly to Jordan, Syria and Lebanon,

according to the U.N. High Commissioner for Refugees. The refugees include large numbers of doctors, academics and other professionals vital for Iraq's recovery. Another 1.7 million have been forced to move to safer towns and villages inside Iraq, and as many as 50,000 Iraqis a month flee their homes, the U.N. agency said in January.

The rich began trickling out of Iraq as conditions deteriorated under UN sanctions in the 1990s, their flight growing in the aftermath of the 2003 U.S.-led invasion. Now, as the violence worsens, increasing numbers of poor Iraqis are on the move, aid officials say. To flee, Iraqis sell their possessions, raid their savings and borrow money from relatives. They ride buses or walk across terrain riddled with criminals and Sunni insurgents, preferring to risk death over remaining in Iraq . . . .

The United Nations is struggling to find funding to assist Iraqi refugees. Fewer than 500 have been resettled in the United States since the invasion. Aid officials and human rights activists say the United States and other Western nations are focused on reconstructing Iraq while ignoring the war's human fallout. (Raghaven, 2007)

Iraq suffers a deterioration of its health care services as physicians flee the country. Poorer refugees strain the resources of their host countries, many suffering a want of basic necessities in refugee camps. Many refugees simply cannot be resettled. This has given rise to a desperate need for nurses for refugee health care—and perhaps an emerging clinical specialization in refugee nursing.

The actions and policies of the United States also affect global health. Ripples in global health spread around the world to reach the United States again. Policies, however, are as much based on ideology as on science. For instance, the Bush administration's policy on HIV/AIDS prevention in Africa is based on an abstinence-only ideology.

The US faces condemnation this week from leaders of the worldwide struggle against AIDS over the Bush administration's reliance on sexual abstinence as a response to the intensifying epidemic. With a major international conference on AIDS being opened by UN Secretary General Kofi Annan today in Bangkok, there are fears that lives are at risk in some of the world's poorest countries because of American objections to a 'safe sex' approach to combating AIDS. Hillary Benn, the UK's International Development Secretary, who spearheads Britain's fight against AIDS overseas, told *The Observer* that an abstinence-only approach would not work. 'We need to have all the means at our disposal to fight the epidemic,' he said. 'People should have access to condoms.' In Brussels, Poul Nielson, the EU's outspoken Commissioner for Development and Humanitarian Aid, criticised America for 'preaching one line only and denying people's rights by trying to push them into abstinence. It will weaken the battle against AIDS, and the unfortunate reality is that it will directly endanger the lives of millions of women.' Under the influence of the Christian right, Bush has adopted the so-called ABC approach to Aids prevention—A for abstinence, B for being faithful and C for condoms. But condoms are to be promoted only for use by 'high risk groups' such as prostitutes and drug abusers, with sexual abstinence the objective for all unmarried young people. Unusually open criticism of US policy has also come from UNAIDS, the UN body responsible for coordinating the global response to AIDS. Dr Peter Piot, executive director, said: 'We know condoms save lives. We are not in the business of morality. Condom promotion should be part of education about sexuality for young people.' Bush's policy was laid down earlier this year in a 100-page document entitled 'The President's Emergency Plan for AIDS Relief'. It is backed by a $15 billion commitment over five years and targets 15 countries, 12 in sub-Saharan Africa. References to condoms—for decades heavily promoted in the US drive for population control in the developing world—make clear that they are to play a marginal role. They can be distributed 'near areas where high-risk behaviour takes place' such as brothels, but they are not to be promoted for the general population, which should receive 'a clear message that the best means of preventing HIV/AIDS is to avoid risk altogether'. (Gill, 2004)

Nonscientific concerns play a substantive role in policy formulation. Just as immigration restrictions and policies have been influenced by eugenic concerns for the American gene pool, foreign aid and policies for AIDS-prevention have been influenced by personal ideology. And health is affected, nationally and worldwide.

There have been worldwide changes in nursing as well. Nurses have "migrated" in large numbers. The reasons for migration are numerous, but include nursing shortages in "destination countries." Table 11.1 shows the international recruitment of nurses. The International Council of Nurses (ICN) has raised a number of issues in nurse migration (Buchan, Kingma, & Lorenzo, 2005).

It is apparent from this ICN chart that a number of moral issues attend nurse migration, not the least of which is the concern for harm to the source country's health care system by the recruitment of their nurses to alleviate a shortage in this country. Many of the source countries are less well developed than the destination countries. What responsibility does a wealthy nation have toward poorer nations? Another major issue is the prejudice faced by foreign-born, foreign-educated nurses. Hirschfield writes that:

. . . poorer countries shoulder the cost of publically financed health professional education and suffer the loss of taxation, loss of work contribution of the migrant person, and loss of health care to the population as a result. Rich countries that recruit human resources from poorer countries thus owe considerable unacknowledged debt to these developing countries. Although remittances provide some compensation for poor countries that 'export' health professionals, these countries will usually experience a net loss of human capital in the health system, with serious implications for quality, coverage and access to services. (Hirschfield, 2006)

TABLE 11.1 International Recruitment of Nurses: Possible Opportunities and Challenges (Buchan, Kingma, & Lorenzo, 2005)

	Opportunities	Challenges
Destination countries	Solve skills/staff shortages. "Quick fix."	How to be efficient and ethical in recruitment.
Source countries	Remittances. Upskilled returners impact on delivery of care. (if they return). Lower unemployment in certain cases.	Outflow may cause shortages; negative impact on delivery of care. Costs of "lost" education. Increased costs of recruitment of replacements "Manage" migration?
Internationally mobile nurses	Improved pay, career opportunities, education.	Achieving equal treatment in destination country.
Static nurses	Improved job and career opportunities (if worker oversupply).	Increased workload as other nurses leave. Lower morale.

Nursing education cannot ignore the consequences of globalization for health or for nursing. It is a moral mandate in today's nursing education.

The world has "gotten smaller." There is no longer any such thing as an isolated health-event that does not affect others. A chicken sold in Korea has the potential to eventually affect the health of a pig or a person in Britain. When you sneeze in New York, a taxi driver in Bangkok catches a cold.

In facing issues that affect global health and global nursing, it is important for nurses to reflect upon questions such as these:

- What is my view of the responsibility of wealthy nations toward poorer and less well-developed nations?
- What is my view of the responsibility of the United States for global health?
- What is my view of the responsibility of the United States for indirect effects upon global health, such as global warming?
- What is my view of war?
- What is my view of ideologically driven national and international health policy?
- What is my attitude toward nurses who immigrate to the United States permanently or temporarily from poorer nations?
- What is my attitude toward hospitals recruiting nurses from other nations and paying them less than prevailing wages and benefits?
- What is my attitude toward nurses who immigrate to the United States in order to send a portion of their salary (a "remittance") to their family in their home country?

CONCLUSION

Two things are critical to note here. First, seemingly unrelated issues—genomics, U.S. demographics, and nursing recruitment—are not, in the end, unrelated. Values suffuse all aspects of our lives, including our nation's policies and realities, and bring seemingly disparate concerns together as if they were but different facets of the same stone. Second, it is important to understand that new issues do not necessarily raise new ethical concerns. New issues are often old moral issues in new garb. That is a good thing–it means that the basic skills developed in ethics as you have studied this text will serve you in the analysis of emerging and as yet unthought-of issues still to come.

Nursing has an admirable and proud history of concern for ethics. It has always forged its own course rather than follow the lead of other professions. From the mid-1870s to the present, nursing has demonstrated an enduring concern for ethics in patient care, in all venues and aspects of nursing, in this nation and around the world. You, the reader, stand in a long line of nurses who have addressed a broad range of ethical issues with courage, perseverance, commitment, intelligence, and compassion; you stand in good company and bear the responsibility to continue and advance this tradition.

Notes

1. http://www.ornl.gov/sci/techresources/ Human_Genome/hg5yp/
2. http://www.theatlantic.com/doc/200106/ shell
3. United States Supreme Court. *Buck v Bell.* 274 US 200 (1927)
4. Ibid.
5. Ibid.
6. http://www.ornl.gov/sci/techresources/ Human_Genome/research/elsi.shtml (accessed on March 24, 2008).
7. US Census Bureau, *United States Census 2000.* http://www.census.gov/main/www/ cen2000.html

References

American Nurses Association. (2001). *Code of ethics for nurses with interpretive statements* (p. 9). Silver Spring, MD: ANA.

Bass, E. J., & Jackson, J. F. (1977). Cerumen types in Eskimos. *American Journal of Physical Anthropology, 47*(2), 209–210.

Brown, L. R. (2001). *Eco-economy: Building an economy for the earth*. Washington, DC: Earth Policy Institute.

Buchan, J., Kingma, M., & Lorenzo, F. M. (2005). *International migration of nurses: Trends and policy implications* (p. 25). Geneva, Switzerland: International Council of Nurses.

D'Adamo, P. (2007). *The geno type diet: Change your genetic destiny to live the longest, fullest, and healthiest life possible*. New York: Broadway.

Davis, A. (2008). Provision two. In M. Fowler (Ed.), *Guide to the code of ethics for nurses: Interpretation and application* (pp. 14–15). Silver Spring, MD: American Nurses Association.

Gibson, C., & Lennon, E. (1999). US Census Bureau, Working Paper No. 29, *Historical Census Statistics on the Foreign-Born Population of the United States: 1850 to 1990*, US Government Printing Office, Washington, DC.

Gill, P. (2004, July 11). Experts attack Bush's stance in AIDS battle. *Guardian,* The Observer/UK. Full Text available: http://observer.guardian.co.uk/print/0,3858,4968385-102275,00.html.

Gould, S. J. (1981). *The mismeasure of man.* New York: Norton.

Hall, E. T. (1989). *Beyond culture.* New York: Anchor Books/Knopf.

Harris, M., & Ross, E. (1987). *Food and evolution: Toward a theory of human food habits.* Philadelphia: Temple University.

Herrnstein, R. (1983). Intelligence tests and the Immigration Act of 1924. *American Psychologist, 38,* 986–995.

Hirschfield, M. (2006). An international perspective. In A. Davis, V. Tschudin, & L. deRaeve (Eds.), *Essentials of teaching and learning in nursing ethics: Perspectives and methods* (p. 326). London: Churchill Livingstone/Elsevier.

Hofstede, G. (2003). *Culture's Consequences: Comparing Values, Behaviors, Institutions and Organizations across Nations* (2nd ed.). Thousand Oaks, CA: Sage.

Lindor, N. M., Lindor, C. J., & Greene, M. H. (2006). Hereditary neoplastic syndromes. In D. Schottenfeld & J. F. Fraumeni, Jr. (Eds.), *Cancer epidemiology and prevention* (3rd ed., pp. 562–576). New York, NY: Oxford University Press.

Martindale, D. (2001, January 18). Pink slip in your genes. *Scientific American.*

Nichols, B. (2007). *Building global alliances III: The impact of global nurse migration on health services delivery.* Philadelphia, PA, USA: Commission on Graduates of Foreign Nursing Schools.

Overfield, T. (1985). *Biologic variation in health and illness: Race, age, and sex differences.* Menlo Park, CA, USA: Addison-Wesley Publishing.

Raghaven, S. (2007, February 4, Sunday). War in Iraq propelling a massive migration. *The Washington Post,* p. A01.

Rothstein, M. (1997). *Genetic secrets: Protecting privacy and confidentiality in the genetic era.* New Haven: Yale University Press.

Scemons, D. (2006). *Words and the Breath of Life.* Prepublication manuscript.

Simpson, J., & Weiner, E. (1989). *The Oxford English Dictionary.* Oxford, UK: Oxford University Press.

UNESCO Universal Declaration on Cultural Diversity. New York: United Nations, 21 February 2002.

United Nations Convention to Combat Desertification. (2004, June 16). *Desertification, Hunger, and Poverty.* Geneva, Switzerland: Institut Universitaire d'Etudes du Dévelopment.

Vernez, G., & McCarthy, K. F. (1997). *Immigration in a changing economy: California's experience.* Santa Monica, CA: The Rand Corporation.

World Health Organization. (1946). *Constitution of the World Health Organization,* Geneva.

World Health Organization. (1986). *The Ottawa Charter for Health Promotion,* Ottawa.

Yoshiura, K. I., Kinoshita, A., Ishida, T., Ninokata, A., Ishikawa, T., Kaname, T., et al. (2006, January 29). A SNP in the ABCC11 gene is the determinant of human earwax type. *Nature Genetics.* DOI:10.1038/ng1733.

APPENDIX

Appendix: Resources

NURSING ETHICS AND BIOETHICS: GENERAL INFORMATION, SELECTED READINGS, AND SELECTED NURSING AUTHORS

ANA

Center for Ethics and Human Rights
Code for Nurses with Interpretative Statements

Other Organizations and Bioethics

1. Hastings Center of Bioethics—Garrison NY
2. Kennedy Center of Ethics
   Kennedy Library of Bioethics
   Georgetown—Washington DC
3. Bioethics Center—University of Penn.
4. Bioethics Center—University of Minn.
5. Institute of Medical Humanities
   University of Texas, Galveston, TX

Online Information

When the first edition of this book was published in 1978, computers were not readily available so each chapter had many references. Now the computer provides multiple sources in bioethics and nursing ethics. As mentioned earlier, it is important to know the source of each of these references and the possible ethical position the writer has taken.

Journals

There is one journal specifically focused on nursing ethics. This journal is the official publication of the International Centre for Nursing Ethics (ICNE) at the University of Surrey, UK. This centre gives Human Rights Awards to nurses annually. It also conducts an annual nursing ethics conference.

Nursing Ethics: An International Journal for Health Care Professionals
Editor—Ann Gallagher, University of Surrey UK
Editor Emerita—Verena Tschudin
 Many other nursing journals publish articles on issues in nursing ethics.
 Non-nursing journals include:

1. *American Journal of Bioethics*
2. *Bioethics*
3. *Cambridge Ethics Quarterly*
4. *Ethics and Medicine: An International Journal of Bioethics*
5. *Eubios Journal of Asian and International Bioethics*
6. *Hastings Center Report*

BACKGROUND READINGS

Selected authors who have written moral philosophy—Aristotle, Kant, Mill, Rawls

Books in Applied Ethics

1. Beauchamp, T. L., & Childress, J. F. (2008). *Principles of biomedical ethics.* New York: Oxford University Press.
2. Davis, A. J., Tschudin, V., & de Raeve, L. (Eds.). (2006). *Essentials of teaching and learning in nursing ethics: Perspectives and methods.* Oxford: Churchill Livingstone.
3. Pinch, W. J. E., & Haddad, A. (2008). *Nursing and health care ethics: A legacy and a vision.* Silver Springs, MD: ANA.
4. Tschudin, V., & Davis, A. J. (Eds.). (2008). *The globalisation of nursing.* Abingdon, Oxford, UK: Radcliffe Medical Press.
5. Fowler, M. (Ed.). (2008). *The guide to the code of ethics for nurses: Interpretation and application.* Silver Spring, MD: American Nurses Association.

Selected Nursing Ethics Authors—USA

Aroskar, Mila
Benner, Patricia
Bishop, Anne
Curtin, Leah
Fry, Sara
Hadad, Amy
Jameton, Andrew
Liaschenko, Joan
Murphy, Catherine
Penticuff, Joy
Pinch, Winifred
Rushton, Cynda
Silva, Mary
Taylor, Carol

INDEX